SpringerBriefs in Public Health

Series Editor
Angelo P. Giardino
Houston, Texas, USA

SpringerBriefs in Public Health present concise summaries of cutting-edge research and practical applications from across the entire field of public health, with contributions from medicine, bioethics, health economics, public policy, biostatistics, and sociology.

The focus of the series is to highlight current topics in public health of interest to a global audience, including health care policy; social determinants of health; health issues in developing countries; new research methods; chronic and infectious disease epidemics; and innovative health interventions.

Featuring compact volumes of 50 to 125 pages, the series covers a range of content from professional to academic. Possible volumes in the series may consist of timely reports of state-of-the art analytical techniques, reports from the field, snapshots of hot and/or emerging topics, elaborated theses, literature reviews, and in-depth case studies. Both solicited and unsolicited manuscripts are considered for publication in this series.

Briefs are published as part of Springer's eBook collection, with millions of users worldwide. In addition, Briefs are available for individual print and electronic purchase.

Briefs are characterized by fast, global electronic dissemination, standard publishing contracts, easy-to-use manuscript preparation and formatting guidelines, and expedited production schedules. We aim for publication 8-12 weeks after acceptance.

More information about this series at http://www.springer.com/series/10138

Sanghamitra M. Misra • Ana Maria Verissimo

A Guide to Integrative Pediatrics for the Healthcare Professional

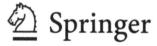 Springer

Sanghamitra M. Misra
Academic General Pediatrics
Baylor College of Medicine
Houston
Texas
USA

Ana Maria Verissimo
Pain and Palliative Care Medicine
Connecticut Children's Medical Centre
Hartford
Connecticut
USA

ISSN 2192-3698   ISSN 2192-3701 (electronic)
ISBN 978-3-319-06834-3   ISBN 978-3-319-06835-0 (eBook)
DOI 10.1007/978-3-319-06835-0
Springer Cham Heidelberg New York Dordrecht London

Library of Congress Control Number: 2014939451

Printed on acid-free paper

Springer is part of Springer Science+Business Media (www.springer.com)

This book is dedicated to our families.
Amit, Veeru, Leelu & Jeevu
Tom, Tommy and Nick
Amy and Sonia

Acknowledgments

We are thankful to the leading integrative pediatricians who opened the doors for us.

A special thank you to Mark Meyer from Baylor College of Medicine for guiding us through the writing process.

Contents

Chapter 1
Introduction to Complementary and Alternative Medicine/Integrative Medicine in Pediatrics

Ana Maria Verissimo and Sanghamitra M. Misra

"It is possible to heal, with your listening, things you cannot cure with your science."

Rachel Naomi Remen, M.D.

The focus of this monograph is the relatively new field of pediatrics known as pediatric integrative medicine (PIM). Integrative medicine (IM) is defined by the Consortium of Academic Health Centers for Integrative Medicine (CAHCIM) as "the practice of medicine that reaffirms the importance of the relationship between practitioner and patient, focuses on the whole person, is informed by evidence, and makes use of all appropriate therapeutic approaches, healthcare professionals and disciplines to achieve optimal health and healing" (CAHCIM 2013). The term complementary and alternative medicine (CAM) is often used interchangeably with IM, but the terms are mutually exclusive. The National Center for Complementary and Alternative Medicine (NCCAM) of the National Institutes of Health (NIH) defines CAM as a group of diverse medical and health care systems, practices, and products that are not presently considered to be part of conventional Western medicine (NCCAM 2013). By definition, complementary medicine is used *in conjunction with* conventional Western medicine, while alternative medicine is used *in place of* conventional Western medicine.

The term CAM does not fully embrace the integration of treatments that is implied in the term IM. IM is the integration of effective CAM therapies into the allopathic practice of medicine. IM practitioners address many facets of a patient's life and utilize effective therapies from many forms of medicine. Figure 1.1 is Collinge's depiction of the spectrum of modalities utilized by an integrative practitioner.

S. M. Misra (✉)
Academic General Pediatrics, Baylor College of Medicine, Houston, TX, USA
e-mail: smisra@bcm.edu

A. M. Verissimo
Pain and Palliative Care Medicine, Connecticut Children's Medical Centre, Hartford, CT, USA
e-mail: averiss@connecticutchildrens.org

S. M. Misra, A. Maria Verissimo, *A Guide to Integrative Pediatrics for the Healthcare Professional,* SpringerBriefs in Public Health, DOI 10.1007/978-3-319-06835-0_1,
© Springer International Publishing Switzerland 2014

1

Fig. 1.1 The integrative medicine wheel. (Reprinted with permission of William Collinge, PhD)

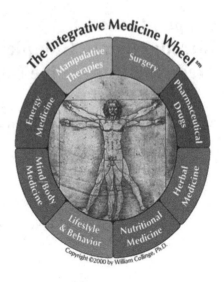

The use of CAM is common among children and adolescents around the world. Specifically in the United States, a national study revealed that approximately 12 % of pediatric patients used CAM therapies in 2007 and CAM use was higher in patients with chronic medical conditions (Barnes et al. 2008). This is important as the pediatric medical landscape has changed dramatically over the last 20 years with an increase in chronic and life-threatening conditions such as asthma, obesity, autism, diabetes, cancer, chronic pain and depression. General knowledge of CAM is becoming crucial for all pediatric practitioners since patients seek non-allopathic treatments, especially for chronic medical conditions. Interestingly, a survey study by Kemper and O'Connor assessing pediatricians who were then active members of the American Academy of Pediatrics (AAP) showed that pediatricians, despite recognizing that many patients were interested in CAM, were not comfortable discussing or recommending such therapies. The survey also delineated that pediatricians were very interested in increasing their knowledge about CAM (Kemper and O'Connor 2004).

Forms of CAM

There are many forms of CAM practiced in the US. For simplicity, the more common forms of CAM are categorized here by systems:

1. Biologically based systems
2. Mind-body practices
3. Manipulative and body-based systems
4. Alternative whole medical systems
5. Energy-based medicine

(1) Biologically Based Systems This includes naturally derived substances such as herbs, foods, vitamins, minerals, and enzymes that are not regulated by the Food and Drug Administration (FDA).

a. Herbal products- used as botanical remedies in the therapeutic treatment of patients
b. Dietary supplements- substances taken orally that have dietary ingredients to supplement the diet

(2) Mind-Body Practices The Mind-Body medicine system utilizes techniques that allow the mind to influence body function.

a. Art/Music/Dance/Aromatherapy: modalities used to create an atmosphere of relaxation, inner peace, and comfort
b. Biofeedback: use of mechanical or electrical devices to reveal physiologic information in response to psychological cues (Culbert and Olness 2010 p. 283)
c. Cognitive Behavioral Therapy (CBT): psychotherapeutic methods used for monitoring, identifying, and transforming thoughts to treat a variety of conditions (Culbert and Olness 2010 p. 527)
d. Diaphragmatic Breathing: relaxation through focused movement of the diaphragm to positively influence the fight-versus-flight response
e. Guided Imagery: a technique of focus on a place or event to create relaxation and comfort
f. Hypnosis: movement to an altered state of awareness and alertness by concentrating on an image or idea with a specific purpose or goal (Culbert and Olness 2010 p. 272)
g. Meditation: the discipline of paying attention, on purpose, without judgment
h. Prayer: a religious form of communication with God, a personal experience
i. Progressive Muscle Relaxation: a relaxation technique of slow tension and subsequent relaxation of various muscle groups
j. Yoga: an ancient Indian practice consisting of postures aligned with breathing, meditation, and concentration in an effort to calm and focus the mind

(3) Manipulative and Body-based Systems These practices involve manipulation of one or more body parts.

a. Chiropractic: based on the interdependence between body structure, usually the spine, and its function in relationship to health and well-being
b. Massage: manipulation of muscle and connective tissue for relaxation
c. Osteopathy: emphasis of disease as manifested through the musculoskeletal system; holds the belief that all the body's systems work together and that which affects one system will then affect another
d. Reflexology: based on the belief that "reflex" areas on the feet and hands are linked to other areas of the body; practitioners apply pressure to reflex areas to assist in health through energetic pathways

(4) Alternative Whole Medical Systems

a. Ayurveda: This 5000-year-old medical practice, which originated in India, emphasizes the importance of the connection between mind, body, and spirit. There is focus on disease prevention. Treatment incorporates nutrition, herbals, exercise, meditation, and yoga.
b. Homeopathy: This practice is founded upon the belief that "like cures like." While high concentrations of a medicinal substance can cause symptoms, an extremely diluted quantity of the same medicinal substance can cure symptoms.
c. Native American Medicine: This system considers the spirit, whose life-force manifestation in humans is called *ni* by the Lakota and *nilch'i* by the Navajo, as an inseparable element of healing. There is emphasis on the *spiritual forces* of the patient, the healer, the patient's family, community, environment, and the medicines themselves. The process of healing takes into account the dynamics among these *spiritual forces* as a part of the universal spirit.
d. Naturopathic Medicine: This system is founded on the belief that there is an innate healing ability within the body. Nutrition, lifestyle choices, exercise, dietary supplements, homeopathy, Traditional Chinese Medicine, and herbals are all utilized in naturopathy.
e. Traditional Chinese Medicine (TCM): This is an ancient system of healthcare from China which incorporates the concept of a vital life force energy known as *qi*. *Qi* is involved in balancing a person's spiritual, emotional, physical, and mental state. *Qi* is influenced by opposing forces that are always in movement, which are represented by *yin* (negative energy) and *yang* (positive energy). When flow of *qi* is disrupted and there is an energy imbalance, disease results. This form of medicine incorporates crucial components such as nutritional support, herbal remedies, exercise, meditation, acupuncture, and massage.

(5) Energy-based Medicine These systems utilize energy fields.

a. Acupuncture/Acupressure: Originating in China as part of TCM, this medical practice is also based on the premise of an essential life force *qi* that flows through meridian lines. When there is an interruption of *qi*, there is disease. The stimulation of the energy points along these lines through the use of needles and/or pressure is believed to improve health.
b. Healing Touch: This therapy is based on the supposition that energy can permeate all matter including layers of the physical body. Any disruption in energy can cause physical, emotional, mental, and spiritual illness. Practitioners use gentle touch to balance the energy for healing (Culbert and Olness 2010 p. 188).
c. Reiki: This therapy, whose name means "Universal Life Energy" in Japanese, is based on the belief that spiritual energy can be channeled through a Reiki practitioner to heal the patient's spirit and physical body.
d. Therapeutic Touch: This is derived from the ancient healing tradition of *laying on* of hands. Therapists detect energy imbalances and influence healing (Culbert and Olness 2010 p. 182).
e. Qi Gong: This practice is a facet of TCM practice whereby movement, meditation, and breathing are used to influence and balance *qi*.

Fig. 1.2 Graph of CAM Use. (Data gathered 2007, Published 2008; http//nccam. nih.gov/news/camstats/2007/ graphics.htm; NOTE: 30–70 % of children with chronic, recurrent and life threatening diseases use some form of CAM; Jean and Cyr 2007; Senser and Kelly 2007, Vol 54)

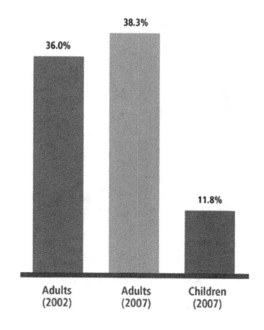

Why People Seek CAM

CAM is sought by patients for a variety of reasons including wellness measures, interest in self-treatment, need for coping strategies, modalities to ease side effects from allopathic treatments, frustration with allopathy, or to utilize a holistic approach to health. Many Westerners are intrigued by the Eastern medical philosophy, which emphasizes a holistic approach toward health care. Patients often seek a sense of control and empowerment over their health and wellness. This drive towards self-care is an important part of IM.

Research has not shown a consistent connection between use of CAM/IM and income, educational level, ethnicity, insurance, age, or gender. It appears that the use of CAM/IM is largely due to interest in seeking care consistent with a person's or family's belief system.

CAM/IM: United States Statistics

In 2007, the NCCAM collected data via the National Health Interview Survey on roughly 24,000 adults and 9400 children (defined as younger than 17 years of age). This information was published by Barnes et al. as a CDC National Health Statistics Report (Barnes et al. 2008).

Figure 1.2 delineates the increase in CAM use among adults in the US from 2002 to 2007 and shows that 11.8 % of children used CAM in 2007. According to two

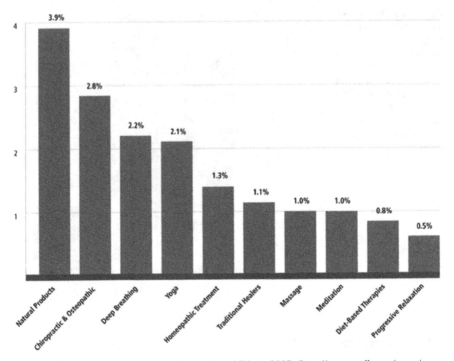

Fig. 1.3 The 10 most common therapies used by children, 2007. (http://nccam.nih.gov/news/cam-stats/2007/graphics.htm)

studies in 2007, 30–70% of children with chronic, recurrent, and life-threatening diseases used some form of CAM (Jean and Cyr 2007; Senser and Kelly 2007).

Overall, it appears that CAM use is growing. The number of CAM providers in the United States is estimated to have increased by 88% between 1994 and 2010. This is in stark contrast with the 16% increase in the number of allopathic or mainstream physicians in the US during this same time period. It is important to note that few CAM providers receive extensive training in pediatrics. Optimal services for efficacy, safety, and research in IM need to align with this change in the overall trend of healthcare.

Figure 1.3 shows the most common therapies used in 2007 among children.

Figure 1.4 delineates the most common natural products used by children in 2007. Echinacea was the most widely used herb.

Figure 1.5 shows that CAM was used by children for acute conditions like the common cold as well as for chronic conditions like ADHD.

Although pediatricians do not always communicate with their patients about CAM, many are knowledgeable about some forms of CAM. A recent study by Kemper showed that greater than 33% of pediatricians reported use of some form of CAM therapy either by themselves and/or a family member, of which 75% used massage, 21% used chiropractic care, 13% used acupuncture, and roughly 13% used spiritual or religious assistance (Kemper et al. 2008).

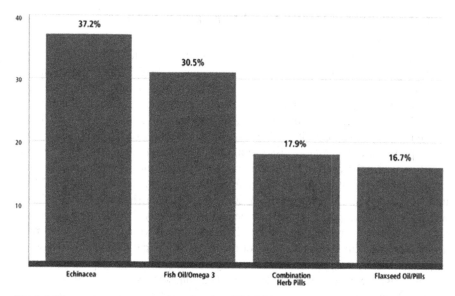

Fig. 1.4 The most common natural products used by children, 2007. (http://nccam.nih.gov/news/camstats/2007/graphics.htm)

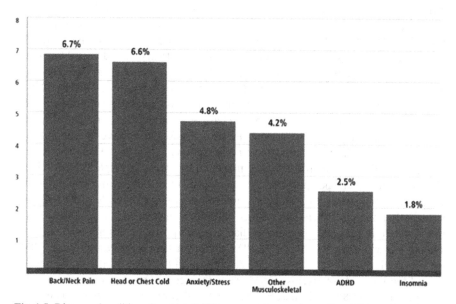

Fig. 1.5 Disesases/conditions for which CAM was most frequently used by children, 2007. (http://nccam.nih.gov/news/camstats/2007/graphics.htm)

Pediatric Chronic Health Conditions and CAM Use

The numbers and types of chronic health conditions in the US are increasing. According to a CDC report from 2013, an estimated 13–20% of children in the United States suffer from mental health disorders within a calendar year and the numbers appear to be increasing. A recent study by Visser et al. showed that 11% of 4–17 year-olds carried a diagnosis of ADHD and 69% of these patients were on medication for this condition. This was an increase of over 28% in medication prescriptions from 2007 data (Visser et al. 2012). According to a 2013 CDC report based on parental report, 4.7% of children (3–17 years old) were diagnosed with anxiety at some point in time. In addition, phobias or fears were estimated at 2.6% in 4–17 year-olds. The estimate from 2001 to 2004 data (NHANES , DISC-IV) was only 0.7% for panic disorder or generalized anxiety disorder in 8–15 year-olds. These trends are alarming (Perou 2013). Children who experience recurrent headaches (migraine or tension-type) or recurrent abdominal pain and who require outpatient tertiary hospital referrals have significant prevalence of psychiatric co-morbidity with anxiety being predominant (Machnes-Maayan et al. 2013). There was a 24% increase in inpatient mental health and substance abuse admissions during a 3-year surveillance study from 2007 to 2010 (Perou 2013).

According to a 2011 CDC study, 14% of children younger than 18 years of age ever had a diagnosis of asthma, 10% still have the diagnosis of asthma, and 19% of children younger than 18 years of age have allergies. Learning disability is estimated at 8% for children 3–17 years old (Bloom et al. 2012). The incidence of childhood obesity has tripled in adolescents and more than doubled in children during the last 30 years (Ogden et al. 2012; NCHS 2011). According to the American Diabetes Association, 1 in 400 US children have diabetes, type 1 or 2 (ADA 2013).

Given the above statistics, a crisis is emerging in the overall health of pediatric patients. There is a demand for preventive care and a greater need for skills to utilize self-regulation and empowerment. Patients desire and deserve an opportunity to participate in their own healthcare and rely less on medications. There is urgency for a multidisciplinary approach to care that embraces these principles. IM provides this unique treatment perspective. The enhancement of developing coping skills and the resulting sense of control and empowerment is the pinnacle of IM. This is particularly important when patients face chronic, recurrent, and/or life-threatening illness. There is concern that many pediatric health professionals are not comfortable talking with patients about CAM/IM, and most families do not discuss CAM use with their allopathic practitioners. According to the 2008 NHIS study, nearly 66% of families did not disclose CAM use to their child's primary care practitioner (Kemper et al. 2008). With increasing numbers of chronic conditions in pediatric patients, allopathic practitioners could benefit from learning about IM. This effort would likely, in turn, benefit patients. Historically in the medical model, patients sought evaluation when symptoms of disease appeared. Over the last 20 years, there has been a shift towards a preventive wellness model in general pediatrics. The specialty of IM broadens this wellness model and can have a significant impact on the health and happiness of the pediatric patient.

Challenges of Integrative Medicine Research

Integrative medicine is comprised of many therapies, and the research behind these therapies is evolving. There are huge limitations in the realm of IM research including financial constraints, concerns about methodology, and product and therapy safety. Possible methodological limitations are especially important for those modalities in which the gold standard of a randomized, double-blind, placebo-controlled study is difficult to execute. In particular, studies with acupuncture, guided imagery and hypnosis, meditation, massage, and yoga may have limitations due to acceptable controls. There are concerns that studies with "sham" acupuncture or "sham" massage therapy cannot have true controls. Often in CAM, the therapy's intervention implies an intrinsic connection between the patient and the provider. This energy exchange may not be *measureable*, but is pertinent. In acupuncture studies, there may be slight variations in depth of penetration of the acupuncture needle, the needle's diameter, the number of needles used, and the length of time the needles are in place. Although the acupuncture points are selected to create a specific outcome in a desired portion of the body, there may be variations in technique from one acupuncturist to another. Massage therapy is another modality in which studies are difficult to standardize as there is slight variation in technique with individual massage treatments. It is difficult to investigate fundamentally different medical systems such as Traditional Chinese Medicine and ayurvedic medicine within a conventional medical model. The allopathic research model may not be effective, as these alternative systems evaluate, diagnose, and treat based on the *Whole Person Model*. The emphasis includes mind, body, and spirit, and focuses on preventive care and a need to diagnose the *root* causes of illness. In this manner, treatment is always individualized. Two patients presenting to an ayurvedic practitioner with the same complaint may leave with the same diagnosis but completely different treatment plans. This makes standardized trials difficult to conduct and results difficult to measure and interpret.

IM studies have been criticized for small sample size, lack of standardization of techniques, and poor data outcome parameters. In addition, the lack of CAM expertise in analyzing these studies may pose inadequate peer review as well as undue restrictions in institutional review board studies.

Children are not *little adults* but are rather unique in their developmental stages and physiological composition. Therefore, data should not be extrapolated from adult studies to form treatment plans for children. It is crucial to promote and conduct pediatric studies of IM. The NCCAM and CAHCIM have been successfully addressing barriers to research in IM especially over the last decade, but this is only a start. Financial constraints affect all areas of research. In 2012, the NIH's total budget was $ 30.9 billion, of which 0.4 % was allocated for NCCAM. In 2006, there were 360 NCCAM-funded research projects. Of this number, less than 5 % were for pediatric research (NCCAM 2013). There are other large sources for financial acquisition like the National Cancer Institute. Most academic and independent hospital centers rely on philanthropy to aid in their research endeavors, and that has been the case for many pediatric IM studies (NCCAM 2013). It is a dynamic time for CAM/IM research, and the growing body of literature will continue to help IM practitioners provide better, more integrated and evidence-based care to their patients.

Reliable Resources This monograph is designed to introduce general pediatric practitioners to the field of integrative pediatrics. It does not include sufficient information for a general practitioner to practice integrative pediatrics. For those interested in further study, refer to the following books and to the reference list at the end of each chapter of this monograph for reliable resources.

- Culbert, Timothy C, Olness, Karen, eds. (2010) Integrative Pediatrics. Oxford University Press. Integrative Medicine Library Series.
- Kemper, Kathi (2010) Mental Health, Naturally. American Academy of Pediatrics.
- Kemper, Kathi (2002) The Holistic Pediatrician. Harper Collins, 2nd edition, HarperQuill.
- Loo, May (2008) Integrative Medicine for Children,1st edition, Saunders.

For practitioners interested in the AAP's recommendations on CAM, please refer to the AAP's section on Integrative medicine and please refer to the following two articles:

- Kemper KJ, Vohra S, Walls R. "The Use of Complementary and Alternative Medicine in Pediatrics: A Clinical Report," *Pediatrics*. Volume 122, Number 6, December 2008, pp. 1374–1368.
- "Recommendations for pediatric clinicians who discuss alternative complementary and unproven therapies with their families" available in the article *Counseling Families Who Choose Complementary and Alternative Medicine for Their Child With Chronic Illness or Disability*. Pediatrics. Vol. 107 No. 3 March 1, 2001, pp. 598–601.

A Medical Timeline with Focus on Pediatrics and CAM

3000 BCE	Ayurveda practiced in India
2000 BCE	Acupuncture practiced in China
300 BCE	Hippocratic Oath emphasizes the entire aspect of the person to understand malady
	Mind-Body-Spirit accepted in medical paradigm
	Belief predominates that imbalance of the four humors (blood, phlegm, yellow, and black bile) causes disease
1641 CE	Rene Descartes' philosophy of dualism emerges-mind and spirit dictated by the church and physical body analyzed by science

1632–1704 CE	John Locke emphasizes rational analysis -all natural phenomena could be reduced to smaller pieces, which added up to create the whole
1796 CE	Hahnemann introduced homeopathy
1840s CE	Popular Health Movement: repeal of laws that forbid alternative practitioners to practice
1847 CE	American Medical Association (AMA) formed to obstruct "alternative medicine" practitioners
1874 CE	Andrew Still introduces osteopathy
1800s (late) CE	20% all practitioners in US are "alternative medicine" practitioners
1890s CE	Palmer introduces chiropractic medicine
1900 CE	AMA lobbies for state licensing laws to reclaim authority over "alternative" providers
1902–1905 CE	Benedict Lust introduces naturopathy/opens first school of naturopathy in New York state
1910 CE	Flexner report shows inconsistencies in medical education in US
1928 CE	Fleming discovers penicillin
1930 CE	American Academy of Pediatrics (AAP) founded
1929 CE	Blue Cross Insurance founded
1948 CE	World Health Organization founded
1952 CE	Inactive polio vaccine introduced by Salk
1960 CE	Ambulatory Pediatric Association founded
1965 CE	Medicaid/Medicare War on Poverty begins
1972 CE	President Nixon visits China with James Reston of New York Times. Reston develops appendicitis, requires appendectomy, and receives acupuncture exclusively for pain relief
1972 CE	Krieger and Kuntz develop Therapeutic Touch -New York University
1978 CE	American Holistic Medical Association founded
1980s CE	Janet Mentgen introduces Healing Touch
1981 CE	First article published on pediatrician burnout
1991 CE	Office of Alternative Medicine established
1993 CE	Eisenberg publishes "Unconventional Medicine in the United States- Prevalence, Cost and Patterns of Use"-34% surveyed used at least one form of CAM in 1990
1996 CE	Kathi Kemper publishes the book "The Holistic Pediatrician"
1998 CE	NIH establishes NCCAM
1999 CE	Consortium of Academic Health Centers for Integrative Medicine (CAH-CIM) established
2005 CE	AAP establishes provisional section of Complementary, Integrative and Holistic Medicine/Section on Complementary and Integrative Medicine (SOCIM)
2008 CE	NCCAM publishes National Health Statistics Report on US CAM use by adults and children (38% and 12%, respectively)
AAP	Clinical Task Force Report on pediatric IM published
2009 CE	Timothy Culbert and Karen Olness publish the book "Integrative Pediatrics"
2013 CE	AAP renames section on Complementary and Integrative Medicine as the "Section on Integrative Medicine"

References

ADA (2013) Data from the 2011 National Diabetes Fact Sheet. http://www.diabetes.org/diabetes-basics/statistics/#sthash.dlBaM53K.dpuf. Accessed 26 Jan 2011

Barnes PM, Bloom B, Nahin R (2008) CDC National Health Statistics Report #12. Complementary and Alternative Medicine Use Among Adults and Children: United States 12:1–23. http://nccam.nih.gov/news/camstats/2007/graphics.htm

Bloom B, Cohen RA, Freeman G (2012) Summary health statistics for U.S. children: National Health Interview Survey, 2011. National Center for Health Statistics. Vital Health Stat 10(254)

Boyd B (2012) Fiscal year budget request statement for the record house subcommittee on Labor Health and Human Services Education Appropriations. Yale's Research Symposium. Josephine Briggs, M.D. Director, NCCAM Budget Request for 2013

Consortium of Academic Health Centers for Integrative Medicine website (2013) http://www.imconsortium.org/about/home.html. Accessed 5 Jan 2014

Culbert T, Olness K (eds) (2010) Integrative Pediatrics. a volume in Integrative Medicine Library (Series—Senior Editor: Andrew Weil). Oxford University Press, New York

Jean D, Cyr C (2007) Use of Complementary and Alternative Medicine in a General Pediatric Clinic. Pediatrics 120:e138–e141

Kemper KJ. Major Medical Developments Prior to the 1900's Adapted from lecture by Kathi Kemper M.D. Wake Forest University and School of Medicine.

Kemper KJ, O'Connor KG (2004) Pediatricians' recommendations for complementary and alternative medical (CAM) therapies. Ambul Pediatr 4(6):482–487

Kemper KJ, Vohra S, Walls R, Task Force on Complementary and Alternative Medicine; Provisional Section on Complementary, Holistic, and Integrative Medicine (2008) American Academy of Pediatrics. The use of complementary and alternative medicine in pediatrics. Pediatrics 122(6):1374–1386

Machnes-Maayan D et al (2013) Screening for psychiatric comorbidity in children with recurrent headache or recurrent abdominal pain. Pediatr Neurol 50:1–8

National Center for Complementary and Alternative Medicine (NCCAM) (2013) http://nccam.nih.gov/health/whatiscam?nav=gsa#integrative. Accessed 6 Jan 2014

Ogden CL et al (2012) CDC childhood obesity fact. Prevalence of obesity and trends in body mass index among US children and adolescents. JAMA 307(5):483–490

Perou R (2013) Mental health surveillance among children in United States 2005–2011. MMWR Surveill Summ 62(2);1–35. http://www.cdc.gov/mmwr. Accessed 3 Jan 2014

Senser S, Kelly K (2007) Complementary and alternative medicine in pediatric oncology. Pediatr Clin N Am 55:1043–1060

Summary Health Statistics for U.S. Children: National Health Interview Survey (2012) Series 10 Number 254

Visser S et al (2012) Trends in the parent-report of health care provider-diagnosed and medicated attention-deficit/hyperactivity disorder: United States, 2003–2011. J Am Acad Child Adolesc Psychiatry 53(1):34–46

Chapter 2
Education

Sanghamitra M. Misra

Complementary and alternative medicine modalities were taught routinely in US medical schools until the early 1900's. In 1908, the Carnegie Foundation for the Advancement of Teaching initiated a survey study of the existing medical schools in the US. The resulting Flexner Report of 1910 forced a sweeping change in medical education and formed a single model of medical education. That model was based on a philosophy that has largely survived to the present day. The Flexner report recommendations forced the removal of CAM education from all allopathic medical schools in the US (Flexner 1910). The reintroduction of CAM into medical student education began largely in the 1990's. In 1995, the Alternative Medicine Interest Group of the Society of Teachers of Family Medicine surveyed U.S. medical school departments of family medicine to determine the extent to which CAM was being taught in medical schools. The results showed that CAM was taught in 34 % of U.S. medical schools (Forjuoh et al. 2003).

An influential movement in CAM education was the NCCAM's CAM Education Project of 1999. The NCCAM initially awarded 14 grants of $ 1–1.5 million to medical schools, teaching hospitals, and the American Medical Student Association (AMSA) to be used for CAM research projects. Over time, CAM has entered the curricula of a growing number of medical schools. The Consortium of Academic Health Centers for Integrative Medicine (CAHIM) is a group of more than 50 U.S. and Canadian medical schools and teaching hospitals that include CAM in their curricula and have CAM focus on at least two of the following: clinical practice, education and research. Medical schools are not training CAM practitioners. The medical school's goal is to expose medical students to the vast array of therapies and medications available to the public. This exposure should be evidence-based and help students learn to promote effective interventions and warn about potentially dangerous interventions.

Introducing medical students to CAM during their training can have lasting effects. Since physicians have the ability to influence politics and society, increasing

S. M. Misra (✉)
Academic General Pediatrics, Baylor College of Medicine, Houston, TX, USA
email: smisra@bcm.edu

S. M. Misra, A. Maria Verissimo, *A Guide to Integrative Pediatrics for the Healthcare Professional,* SpringerBriefs in Public Health, DOI 10.1007/978-3-319-06835-0_2,
© Springer International Publishing Switzerland 2014

awareness of CAM on a political level by physicians can increase funding for CAM research and eventually lead to improved delivery of integrated healthcare. On an ethical level, physicians can push for removal of products or warnings to decrease consumer expenditure on unproven medications and therapies. With increasing positive evidence, health insurance companies can potentially reimburse for more CAM therapies. On a legal level, increased awareness can lead to creation of best-practice guidelines. And, there can be a push for structured and consistent education and licensure for CAM providers. With increased coverage of CAM in medical schools across the US, collaborations can improve overall research and educational curricula (Mills et al. 2002). In a pilot study by Frenkel et al., the authors showed that "integrating CAM into the medical school curriculum requires a dedicated team if it is to result in a significant change. This change requires that CAM practices are visible to both students and faculty, that there is a co-operative climate, accessible resources, and institutional support, and that CAM content is embedded into the existing curriculum"(Frenkel et al. 2007). Many medical schools have initiated Integrative Medicine departments that include IM clinics, IM education and IM research. More than 20 medical schools in the US offer an IM clinic elective for fourth-year students. A number of medical schools have combined the Integrative Medicine department with the department of "wellness" for medical students, residents and faculty while others have a dedicated "wellness" initiative.

According to Vohra et al., "Pediatric integrative medicine (PIM) is emerging as a new subspecialty to better help address twenty-first century patient concerns" (Vohra et al. 2012). Residency is an important place to offer PIM education. As residents learn about clinical practice in their field, it is important for training programs to introduce basic concepts of IM alongside traditional training. More than 20 residency programs in the US offer electives in IM, but most are not pediatrics-focused. At this time, there are no accredited residencies or fellowships in integrative pediatrics. The University of Arizona has instituted a unique online education curriculum for Pediatric Integrative Medicine in Residency (PIMR). PIMR was launched there in October 2012 as a pilot program with 100 h of education. Participants beginning July 2013 also included the University of Kansas, University of Chicago, Eastern Virginia Medical School/Children's Hospital of the King's Daughters and Stanford University. In December 2013, Ohio State University's Center for Integrative Health and Wellness launched an online program for health professionals providing evidence-based training on herbs and supplements.

The American Academy of Pediatrics has a dedicated Section of Integrative Medicine (SOIM), which was established to develop and identify educational opportunities and to advocate for research on complementary and alternative therapies used in pediatrics. According to the American Board of Physician Subspecialties, approximately 25 fellowships in Integrative Medicine are approved by the American Board of Integrative Medicine. Overall, there is a trend to increase awareness and education of IM in medical training (IOM 2005).

References

Flexner A (1910) Medical Education in the United States and Canada: a report to the Carnegie Foundation for the Advancement of Teaching, Bulletin No. 4. New York City: The Carnegie Foundation for the Advancement of Teaching, p 346, OCLC 9795002. Accessed 12 March 2013

Frenkel M, Frye A, Heliker D et al (2007) Lessons learned from complementary and integrative medicine curriculum change in a medical school. Med Educ 41(2):205–213

Forjuoh SN, Rascoe TG, Symm B et al (2003) Teaching medical students complementary and alternative medicine using evidence-based principles. J Altern Complement Med 9(3):429–439

IOM (Institute of Medicine) (2005) US Committee on the Use of Complementary and Alternative Medicine by the American Public. Complementary and alternative medicine in the United States. National Academies Press (US), Washington, DC; Educational Programs in CAM. http://www.ncbi.nlm.nih.gov/books/NBK83809. Accessed 3 Dec 2013

Mills EJ, Hollyer T, Guyatt G et al (2002) Teaching evidence-based complementary and alternative medicine. 1. A learning structure for clinical decision changes. J Altern Complement Med 8(2):207–214.

Vohra S et al (2012) Pediatric integrative medicine: pediatrics' newest subspecialty? BMC Pediatr 12:123

Chapter 3
Modalities of Complementary and Alternative Medicine

Sanghamitra M. Misra, Richard J. Kaplan and Ana Maria Verissimo

I. Acupuncture

Background Acupuncture, a classical form of Traditional Chinese Medicine (TCM), is a collection of procedures involving penetration of the skin with needles to stimulate certain points on the body to create a desired outcome (NCCAM 2013). The concept of acupuncture was widely introduced to the United States in 1971 when New York Times reporter James Reston wrote about his trip to China during which he underwent appendectomy and doctors successfully used needles for pain control. Acupuncture has since become a widely utilized therapy for a variety of conditions in the US. In acupuncture, it is believed that stimulating specific points on the body with small needles corrects imbalances in the flow of *qi* through channels known as meridians. Correcting imbalance can lessen symptoms of pain or disease. Per Dr. Yin Lo (2004),

- *Qi* is vibration.
- *Qi* is oscillation of the meridians.
- *Qi* is what carries the effect of acupuncture from one acupoint to other parts of the body.

From the National Health Statistics Survey of 2007, an estimated 3.1 million U.S. adults and 150,000 children had used acupuncture in the previous year (Barnes et al. 2008a, b). In a survey of parents of children with developmental disorders, 3 % used

S. M. Misra (✉)
Academic General Pediatrics, Baylor College of Medicine, Houston, TX, USA
e-mail: smisra@bcm.edu

R. J. Kaplan
Texas Center of Integrative Medicine, PLLC, Dallas, USA
e-mail: Rich.Kaplan@gmail.com

A. M. Verissimo
Pain and Palliative Care Medicine, Connecticut Children's Medical Centre, Hartford, CT, USA
e-mail: averiss@connecticutchildrens.org

S. M. Misra, A. Maria Verissimo, *A Guide to Integrative Pediatrics for the Healthcare Professional*, SpringerBriefs in Public Health, DOI 10.1007/978-3-319-06835-0_3,
© Springer International Publishing Switzerland 2014

acupuncture or moxibustion and 57% of parents intended to use these therapies in the future (Kim et al. 2013). Moxibustion is a TCM technique that involves the burning of a spongy herb, known as mugwort, to facilitate healing. Moxibustion may be performed with acupuncture needles. Families visit acupuncturists on their own, but allopathic physicians are also beginning to recommend this therapy. A survey study of children presenting to an integrative pediatric clinic with complaints of pain showed that 24% were referred to acupuncture specialists (Young and Kemper 2013).

Basics Acupuncture is the stimulation of specific points on the surface of the skin which have the ability to alter various biochemical and physiological conditions to achieve a desired effect. It is believed that acupuncture points are areas of designated electrical sensitivity and by inserting needles at these points, a practitioner can stimulate various sensory receptors that stimulate nerves. These nerves then transmit impulses to the hypothalamic-pituitary system at the base of the brain which results in the desired effect, often decreasing pain (Joswick 2014).

Evidence Treating pain is a common motivation for utilizing acupuncture. A recent study showed that acupuncture decreases perceived pain in children and adolescents after tonsillectomy (Ochi 2013). Studies in children also show usefulness of acupuncture in a variety of non-pain related conditions. One study looking at enuresis concluded that in patients with primary nocturnal enuresis, acupuncture appears effective in increasing the percentage of dry nights, with continuing results after the end of treatment (El Koumi et al. 2013). Focusing on asthma, one study showed that low-intensity laser acupuncture can be a safe and effective treatment in asthmatic children (Elseify et al. 2013). Laser acupuncture uses laser light in place of needles but stimulates the traditional points mapped by TCM. In a Danish study, acupuncture showed positive effects on asthma in preschool children during treatment, but not after the end of treatment, as assessed by subjective parameters and use of medication (Karlson and Bennicke 2013). In a study of 40 children with perennial allergic rhinitis, there was significant improvement of symptoms with treatment using LED phototherapy and laser acupuncture. Both treatments were considered to be safe (Moustafa et al. 2013).

Safety Relatively few complications have been reported from the use of acupuncture, but potentially serious side effects are possible if not delivered properly by a qualified practitioner (NCCAM 2013). In a systematic review of pediatric acupuncture, the majority of adverse events associated with pediatric needle acupuncture were mild in severity. Many of the serious adverse events were likely a result of substandard practice. It is extremely important that children receive acupuncture services from qualified and experienced acupuncturists (Adams et al. 2011).

Education In the US, there are approximately 50 accredited acupuncture schools. The Accreditation Commission for Acupuncture and Oriental Medicine (ACAOM), founded in 1982 by the Council of Colleges of Acupuncture and Oriental Medicine and the American Association of Oriental Medicine, is recognized by the U.S. Department of Education as a *specialized and professional accrediting* agency, The ACAOM accredits programs and institutions that meet their requirements.

A complete list of accredited programs is available at the website http://www. acaom.org/find-a-school/ (ACAOM 2014).

II. Aromatherapy

Background Aromatherapy is the use of volatile plant materials, known as essential oils, and other aromatic compounds to improve an individual's physical, emotional, and spiritual well-being. Essential oils can be absorbed through the skin and travel through the bloodstream to have effects on the whole body. Distilled essential oils have been employed as medicines since the invention of distillation in the eleventh century (Forbes 1970). Many such oils are described by Roman physician Dioscorides, along with beliefs of the time regarding healing properties of herbs, in his De Materia Medica, written in the first century (Goodyer et al. 1959). Numerous essential oils are available in the US market, each with its own healing properties. According to a study of outpatient pediatric practices in 2013, aromatherapy was one of the top 4 types of CAM used (Adams et al. 2013). Interestingly, a pilot study in 2008 demonstrated that children have specific essential oil scent preferences that may be based on gender and ethnicity (Fitzgerald et al. 2007).

Basics The three modes of aromatherapy include:

- *Aerial diffusion* generally used for:
  - environmental fragrancing
  - disinfection
- *Direct inhalation* generally used for:
  - respiratory disinfection
  - decongestion/expectoration
  - to stimulate brain function
  - to create psychological effects
- *Topical applications* generally used for:
  - therapeutic skin care
  - whole-body healing through compresses or massage

Evidence Studies of aromatherapy do not consistently show benefit. Some essential oils such as tea tree have demonstrated antimicrobial effects, but there is still a lack of clinical evidence demonstrating efficacy against bacterial, fungal, or viral infections (Carson et al. 2006). In general, there is some evidence that essential oils may have therapeutic potential (Edris 2007). A study in adolescents showed that aromatherapy *was* a useful tool in crisis management (Fowler 2006). A pilot study in children with autism in a residential school setting did not show sleep pattern benefit from lavender oil therapy (Williams 2006). Aromatherapy is an option in Rett syndrome (Lotan 2007). Massage with essential oils/aromatherapy is ineffective for childhood eczema (Yates et al. 2007). However, aromatherapy may help with the itching related to eczema (Stein et al. 2012). Children's distress in a perianesthesia setting may be improved with lavender and ginger essential oils (Nord and Belew 2009). Aromatherapy massage seems to reduce hospitalized pediatric burn patients' distress (O'Flaherty 2012). In a 2011 study, inhalation of a mixture of essential oils resulted in a 42.5 % decrease of acute respiratory illnesses and rhinitis (Kilina and Kolesnikova 2011). One trial did not demonstrate benefit of inhalation aromatherapy with bergamot essential oil for reducing anxiety, nausea, or pain in children undergoing stem cell infusion (Ndao et al. 2012). A Korean study showed that abdominal meridian massage with aroma oils (AMMAO) is an effective intervention in relief of constipation for hospitalized children with disability involving the brain (Nam et al. 2013). Aromatherapy with natural essential oil of orange could reduce anxiety during dental procedures (Jafarzadeh et al. 2013).

Safety Safety testing on essential oils shows very few serious side effects when used as directed. Lavender and tea tree oils have hormone-like effects and should be used with caution (NCI 2013). Aromatherapy should be used with caution in children, especially young children, as oils may irritate the skin. There is also a risk of accidental ingestion if children are not monitored properly around essential oils.

Education There are five recognized schools and one nationally accredited school of aromatherapy in the United States. The Alliance of International Aromatherapists (AIA) maintains a list of the available educational programs in the US and Canada (AIA 2013). The National Association for Holistic Aromatherapy (NAHA) is an educational, nonprofit organization that has established education guidelines for aromatherapy (NAHA 2013).

Licensing of practitioners Aromatherapy practitioners are not licensed in the United States. Licensed health professionals such as physicians, nurses, and counselors who have training in aromatherapy may provide the service. The Aromatherapy Registration Council registers practitioners who have passed a national exam and their website (http://aromatherapycouncil.org/) provides a list of aromatherapy practitioners for patients searching for a practitioner near their home.

III. Ayurveda

Background Ayurveda is a form of traditional medicine that originated in India and has been practiced continuously for over 5000 years. Its early history was largely an oral tradition passed from one generation to the next by local healers. Between 1500 and 2000 years ago, Ayurveda was codified into three main texts: one medical, one surgical, and one a composite of the two. These texts were written in Sanskrit and contain healing measures for physical, mental, spiritual, and paranormal insults. Ayurveda is a Sanskrit word composed of the root *Ayur* meaning life and *veda* meaning science. Together, these create "Ayurveda"—the science of life. Like other holistic medical systems, Ayurveda focuses on the connection between mind, body, and spirit.

Basics Ayurvedic philosophy seeks to understand the real-time well being of an individual. It approaches this task with a qualitative system of measurement called *doshas*. In Ayurveda, the three *doshas* of *vata, pitta, and kapha* are believed to control and organize the world from the smallest cell up through the seasons, weather, and time of day. By utilizing a qualitative description of the universe, Ayurveda approaches the complex task of determining how an individual interfaces with the world around him. Diet, sleep/wake times, eating times, sensory stimulus, thought, emotion, season, and climate all play a role in modifying the body's *doshas*.

The three *doshas* of Ayurveda each have specific qualities associated with them. These qualities are called *gunas* and like the Chinese system of *yin* and *yang*, they consist of paired opposites. Some examples of *gunas* are hot and cold, rough and smooth, dry and oily, sharp and dull. With this organization, one can discern the effect of one object on another, even if the effect is subtle. Consider for instance the effect of alcohol on the body. In Ayurveda, alcohol would be assigned the qualities of hot (it warms and causes flushing), penetrating (it is readily absorbed), and subtle (it is rather ethereal in effect). As such, when consumed, it imparts these qualities to the body. In the cold of winter, these qualities, being opposite to the climate, may improve the health of an individual if taken in moderation. In the summer, on the other hand, this additional heat may have detrimental effects.

Each *dosha* is related to a basic force of nature, and has qualities similar to that force. *Vata* is considered akin to the wind, and like the wind it possesses qualities that are drying, rough, mobile, light, and subtle. *Pitta* is considered akin to fire, and as such, it is hot, sharp, penetrating, and slightly mobile. *Kapha* is considered most akin to earth and is nurturing, stable, dull, and cool. In health, each *dosha* serves several specific purposes. *Vata* is said to create movement in the body including the transmission of nerve impulses, the coursing of blood through veins and arteries, and the movement of air with inhalation and exhalation. *Pitta*, the power of transformative change, is believed to serve the metabolic purposes of the body including the digestion of food, maintenance of body temperature, the work of enzymes, and the spark of intelligence and focus. Finally, *Kapha*, the stabilizing force, is said to give foundation and structure to the body including maintaining the health of bones, the lubrication of joints, and the storage of memory. Ayurveda believes that the three *doshas* are in constant flux. Each moment, the strength of each *dosha* within an individual changes based on the environment around the individual. Diet, lifestyle choices, sensory stimuli, emotion, thought, and environmental factors like season and time of day push and pull the *doshas*. If the environment possesses qualities similar to a particular *dosha*, then that *dosha* will increase. Similarly, if the environment possesses qualities dissimilar to a particular *dosha*, then that *dosha* will decrease. Thus, to approach the health of an individual, one must understand two important factors: the baseline constitution of that individual and that individual's current *doshic* state.

In Ayurveda, the baseline constitution of an individual is called *Prakruti*. *Prakruti* is the unique proportion of *vata, pitta, and kapha* that serves as the baseline or balanced state of an individual. *Prakruti* is imparted at conception and can be considered most akin to a combination of genetic predisposition and personality.

Prakruti orients a person to the world, determining strengths and weaknesses, likes and dislikes, and physical, emotional, and psychologic attributes. *Prakruti* can be measured by Ayurvedic practitioners through a combination of pulse diagnosis and appearance. While *Prakruti* tells us the baseline constitution of an individual, *Vikruti* tells us the quantity of the three *doshas* at any given moment. As individuals constantly engage with the world, their internal chemistry, psychology, and emotions constantly shift. Some stimuli push people towards their balance, and others push them away. As each individual is built differently, the same two stimuli may have different effects on an individual depending on their *Prakruti* or baseline nature. When healthy, *Prakruti* and *Vikruti* are closely aligned. As imbalance arises, through the myriad stimuli that the body and mind experience each day, the proportions of *vata, pitta, and kapha* in an individual move away from their baseline state. This can result in small changes in a person's health—constipation, insomnia, indigestion, or other seemingly small problems that are transient and rarely result in a visit to a physician. If these imbalances are not corrected, Ayurveda believes that deeper issues occur and full blown illness can result.

Pediatrics, or *child life*, is one of the major divisions of Ayurveda. The Ayurvedic pediatrician's role begins at conception and continues until the child reaches the age of 16 years (Athavale 2013). The approach to a pediatric patient is similar to that of an adult patient, but treatments tend to be tempered in strength and duration so as not to adversely impact a developing system.

Traditionally, pulse diagnosis is the centerpiece of an Ayurvedic examination. From the pulse alone, experienced practitioners are able to determine *Prakruti, Vikruti*, and the functioning of the patient's physiologic system and main vital organs. Additionally, practitioners may use the tongue, iris, and physical appearance of an individual as well as a more modernly traditional history and physical. Special attention is typically paid to the digestive health of each patient. Improper digestion and elimination is considered one of the earliest signs of imbalance. Restoring regular hunger, proper digestion, and effortless elimination is believed to greatly aid the overall health of the body. Ayurvedic treatments are greatly diverse but a modifications in diet, eating times, and lifestyle habits tend to be the centerpiece of intervention. Additionally, herbal remedies, oil preparations, steam, heat, mantras, ceremony, physical exercise, and enema may all be utilized to restore balance.

As an example, in a child suffering from allergic rhinitis, an Ayurvedic practitioner may make a variety of suggestions:

- **Diet**: Restrict of heavy, sticky (*kapha*) foods including cheese, milk, yogurt, icecream, peanut butter, cream sauces, ripe bananas, mangos, dates, and figs. Use heating spices in food including black pepper, cumin, salt, chili powder, etc.
- **Lifestyle**: Eliminate late night meals, ensure regular/proper eating times, ensure regular/proper sleep/wake times, reduce "sleeping in" and naps, promote exercise and physical exertion
- **Cleansing**: Sauna treatment for dry heat; Sunning for heat; Ensure regular bowel movements
- **Herbal treatment**: Gentle, clearing herbs that are heating such as Zingiber officinale (ginger)

Evidence As Ayurveda involves nuanced treatment unique not only to the individual, but also to the current state of that particular individual, it is difficult to apply double-blind placebo-controlled studies to Ayurvedic treatment methods. Accordingly, although significant anecdotal evidence exists for the utility of Ayurveda, there is little conclusive evidence as to its efficacy in clinical trials and systematic reviews. The body of evidence in Ayurveda, however, is growing. A study of 123 children in India concluded that Trikatrayadi Lauha is significantly effective in the management of iron deficiency anemia in children (Kumar and Garai 2012). A review article of Ayurvedic treatment of children with dyslexia concluded that Ayurveda can treat dyslexia by balancing doshas and providing Medhya drugs that promote intellect (Sharma et al. 2012). However, a subsequent article warned that Ayurveda may be an acceptable adjunct therapy but remedial education is vital for a child's success (Karande and Sholapurwala 2013). Sridharan et al. conducted a review of studies of Ayurvedic herbal medications for diabetes mellitus in children. The group concluded that, "Although there were significant glucose-lowering effects with the use of some herbal mixtures, due to methodological deficiencies and small sample sizes we are unable to draw any definite conclusions regarding their efficacy." There were no significant adverse events reported (Sridharan 2011). One randomized double-blind placebo-controlled trial including 75 adults given either Tinospora cordifolia (TC) or placebo for 8 weeks showed that TC significantly decreased all symptoms of allergic rhinitis. Nasal smear cytology and leukocyte count correlated with clinical findings. TC was well-tolerated (Badar et al. 2005). TC has not been studied in children.

Safety Ayurveda is a complicated discipline that should be practiced only by trained practitioners. Ayurvedic interventions tend to be subtle and gentle, but some treatments, especially herbal, enema, and the clearing methods of *Panchakarma* can cause significant harm to patients if used inappropriately. Ayurveda also uses many metals in the treatment of patients including lead, mercury, gold, and silver. Though these are extensively and precisely processed so as not to cause harm, they are considered very risky treatments in the United States. As such, safety concerns have also been raised about Ayurveda. The FDA issued an alert in 2008 after two concerning studies (Saper et al. 2004). A 2004 study showed that 20 % of Ayurvedic "herbal medicine products" produced in South Asia and available in South Asian grocery stores in Boston contained potentially harmful levels of lead, mercury, and/or arsenic (Saper et al. 2008). The second study in 2008 showed that one-fifth of U.S.-manufactured and Indian-manufactured Ayurvedic products bought on the Internet contained detectable lead, mercury, or arsenic (Valiathan 2006). In addition, a case report was published in 2013 of a 2-year-old girl in India who developed anuric renal failure from chronic ingestion of an Ayurvedic medicine containing mercury (Sathe et al. 2013). That being said, a number of Ayurvedic herbs are now grown in the US and American practitioners can procure herbs from US-based companies. Practitioners and patients may be more informed about the safety of these American products.

Education In India, Ayurvedic training is a 4 to 6 year program. In the United States there are a few schools that offer training of between 400 and 800 classroom hours. This usually takes 9–15 months. Unless additional hands-on or guided training is given, practitioners emerging from these schools are often less equipped to practice Ayurveda than those that have extensive training in India.

Licensing of Practitioners The United States does not have a licensing body for Ayurvedic practitioners. There are organizations that Ayurvedic practitioners can join such as the American Holistic Medical Association, the Integrative Medicine and Holistic Health Association, and the National Ayurvedic Medical Association.

IV. Biofeedback

Background Biofeedback is the process in which a person gains awareness of his/her physiological functions using instruments to provide information on the activity of systems with the goal of being able to manipulate these functions at will (Durand and Barlow 2009). Electronic or mechanical equipment is used to measure physiologic functions, but equipment is not necessarily required to practice biofeedback. Biofeedback is used widely to improve a variety of health conditions. When equipment is used, various physiologic parameters are measured including muscle tension, surface blood flow, heart rate, sweat or galvanic skin response, diaphragmatic breathing, and brain waves (via EEG). Hand-held devices that are available for home use primarily measure heart rate variability. Biofeedback devices objectively record physiologic changes in a non-invasive manner, which a patient can use to gain understanding of the mind-body connection. Hans Selye, MD, a pioneer in stress studies, demonstrated the significant influence stress has on physical and mental health conditions. His early research led to the importance of relaxation strategies to promote homeostatic balance. Dr. Selye laid the foundation for Mind-Body Medicine (Culbert and Olness 2010).

Basics Focusing on subtleties of physiologic functions is the key to the practice of biofeedback. Biofeedback helps patients gain better mind-body appreciation and inner control. Biofeedback utilizes diaphragmatic breathing by emphasizing abdominal rise and fall with minimal movement of the upper chest. Inspiration and expiration is taught to occur through the nose while the patient is *noticing* the sensation. The overall goal is to increase the volume of the breath and decrease the respiratory rate. In thermal biofeedback, blood flow is indirectly measured. The goal is to achieve vasodilation at the capillary level by relaxing smooth muscle and *quieting* the sympathetic nervous system. In biofeedback focusing on muscle tension, electromyography (EMG) measurements are taken by placing electrodes on nonspecific muscle to assess general muscle tension, and then electrodes are placed on specific areas of pain or tension to measure the difference in tension. Biofeedback using heart rate variability is an indicator of autonomic nervous system (ANS) balance. This is an advanced technique usually measured after the patient has familiarity with biofeedback. A greater awareness of one's body allows for "voluntary" control over emotional and physiologic response and allows for balance of the ANS and central nervous system (CNS). Patients learn how to identify and control their psycho-physiologic response to external stimuli. Positive thoughts, like appreciation and caring, can improve balance within the ANS while negative thoughts and emotions contribute to imbalance within the ANS. Biofeedback is usually taught in 4–6 1-h sessions. Home practice increases overall biofeedback competency and efficacy.

Evidence The literature supporting biofeedback for pain control is extensive. In a study of adults with migraine and tension-type headache, biofeedback showed significant benefit (Nestoriuc et al. 2008). According to Tan et al., "Sufficient meta-analysis, detailed reviews, assessments by U.S. government sponsored panels, and high quality studies with long follow ups of significant numbers of patients have demonstrated that biofeedback can be efficacious for assessing and treating a variety of disorders characterized by pain" (Tan et al. 2007). A meta-analysis concluded that neurobiofeedback treatment can be beneficial in patients with attention-deficit/hyperactivity disorder (ADHD) as it was highly effective for patients with inattention and impulsivity and was moderately effective for patients with hyperactivity (Arns et al. 2009). Gevensleben et al. also found neurofeedback to be beneficial in patients with ADHD (Gevensleben et al. 2009). A study published in 2014 showed that an elementary school-based teacher-led daily stress management intervention with biofeedback measurements can decrease anxiety and improve relaxation (Bothe et al. 2014). A study focusing on bowel and bladder dysfunction in children with vesiculoureteral reflux demonstrated that biofeedback is a reasonable therapy (Elder and Diaz 2013). Biofeedback, by increasing sphincter pressure, was also found to be useful in improving anorectal function in children with fecal incontinence (Ambartsumyan and Nurko 2013).

Safety According to the American Cancer Society, "Biofeedback is thought to be a safe technique. It is noninvasive and requires little effort. There have been occasional reports of dizziness, anxiety, disorientation, and a sensation of floating, which may be emotionally upsetting to some people. Biofeedback requires a trained and certified professional to manage equipment, interpret changes, and monitor the patient. Battery-operated devices sold for home use have not been found to be reliable" (ACS 2013).

Education Regionally accredited institutions in the United States and Europe have adopted the Biofeedback Certification International Alliance (BCIA) Blueprints of Knowledge for standardization. There are currently 13 accredited schools of biofeedback in the US. Sources listed below have information regarding training and product information:

- www.bcia.org
- www.heartmath.com
- www.aapb.org
- www.stresseraser.com

- www.stens-biofeedback.com
- www.wildDivine.com

Licensing of Practitioners The Biofeedback Certification International Alliance (BCIA), formerly known as the Biofeedback Institute of America, was created in 1981 with the primary mission of certifying individuals who meet education and training standards in biofeedback and progressively recertifying those who advance their knowledge through continuing education (BCIA 2013). Professionals certified by BCIA in General Biofeedback may refer to themselves as Board Certified in Biofeedback (BCB), in Neurofeedback as Board Certified in Neurofeedback (BCN), and in Pelvic Muscle Dysfunction Biofeedback as Board Certified in Biofeedback for Pelvic Muscle Dysfunction (BCB-PMD) (Schwartz and Montgomery 2003). Individual insurance plans vary, but some insurance companies now cover biofeedback. Practitioners should provide relevant research data regarding biofeedback to their patients and insurance companies to advocate for treatment when appropriate.

V. Biofield Therapies

Biofield therapies are based on the interactions of the human energy field with a greater universal healing energy. Energy therapies are those involving the manipulation of subtle biofield energy to facilitate the body's innate natural healing. Energy medicine's foundation is based on the premise that changes in the *life force* of the body impact health (NCCAM 2013). These forces include electric, magnetic, and electromagnetic fields. Veritable energy fields are mechanical vibrations and electromagnetic forces which use specific, measurable wavelengths and frequencies to treat patients. Implicit to the biofields is that humans have a subtle energy which is currently immeasurable. Examples of biofield include the *qi* in Traditional Chinese Medicine and *doshas* in ayurvedic medicine.

To date, there is no scientific consensus regarding mechanism of action of energy therapies (NCCAM 2013). Practitioners of energy medicine believe that illness results from blockages of these subtle energies. Acupuncture and acupressure work on the belief that diagnosing and restoring the imbalances of the biofield enables the proper flow of *qi*, which in turn restores balance and health. Some therapists are believed to transmit vital energy to a recipient to restore health. The four common biofield therapies are acupuncture, Reiki, healing touch, and therapeutic touch.

VI. Chiropractic

Background The term "chiropractic" combines the Greek words *cheir* (hand) and *praxis* (practice) to describe a treatment done by hand. Hands-on therapy, especially adjustment of the spine, is central to chiropractic care, which is based on the notion that the manner in which a body's structure connects to its function affects an individual's health (NCCAM 2013), The goal of spinal and joint manipulation is to correct alignment problems, alleviate pain, improve function, and support the body's natural ability to heal itself. Although joint manipulation is mentioned in Chinese and Greek texts dating back to 2700 BCE, the chiropractic profession officially began in 1895, when magnetic healer Daniel David Palmer restored the hearing of Harvey Lillard by manually adjusting his neck. In 1897, Dr. Palmer established the Palmer School of Chiropractic in Davenport, Iowa.

According to the 2007 National Health Interview Survey (NHIS), about 8 % of adults (more than 18 million) and nearly 3 % of children (more than 2 million) had received chiropractic or osteopathic manipulation in the preceding 12 months (NC-CAM 2013). Also in 2007, a survey of pediatric patients in an outpatient facility showed that 19 % of the families sought chiropractic care for their children (Jean and Cyr 2007). A study in 2008 showed that approximately 14 % of chiropractic patients are children under 18 (Council on Chiropractic Education 2007). A recent study in Canada showed that almost 28 % of cancer patients in two children's hospitals visited chiropractors (Valji et al. 2013).

Basics Chiropractic is based on the connections between the nervous system and musculoskeletal system. Chiropractors believe that malalignment of joints causes pain and disease. Chiropractors perform adjustments to realign joints. When chiropractors perform adjustments in children, they generally use less force and often utilize a tool known as an *activator*. Chiropractors are generally associated with one of two groups (Lee et al. 2000). Neither group supports routine childhood vaccination. The International Chiropractic Association, established by Dr. Palmer in 1926, promotes chiropractic as essential to health promotion and "is supportive of a conscience clause or waiver in compulsory vaccination laws, providing an elective course of action for all regarding immunization" (ICA 2013). The American Chiropractic Association, founded in 1922, provides more focused treatment on musculoskeletal disorders but also supports autonomy "by maintaining an individual's right to freedom of choice in health care matters and providing an alternative elective course of action regarding vaccination" (ACA 2009). Despite this difference in vaccine belief between allopathic pediatricians and chiropractors, Vallone et al. state that "chiropractors may assume the role of primary care for families who are pursuing a more natural and holistic approach to health care for their families" (Vallone et al. 2010).

Evidence Although the most common reason pediatric patients visit chiropractors is spinal pain, no adequate studies have been performed in this area (Hestbaek and Stochkendahl 2010). The efficacy of chiropractic care in the treatment of nonmusculoskeletal disorders has yet to be definitely proven or disproven (Ferrance and Miller 2010). A review study showed potential benefit in children with respiratory illnesses with manual therapies such as osteopathy, massage, and chiropractics (Pepino et al. 2013). There may be benefit of chiropractic in children with ballistic tremors (Alcantara and Adamek 2012). One case study showed potential benefit of spinal manipulation therapy (SMT) for children with attention deficit hyperactivity disorder (ADHD) (Muir 2012), but a systematic review from 2010 concluded that at that time, there was insufficient evidence to evaluate the efficacy of chiropractic care for pediatric and adolescent ADHD (Karpouzis et al. 2010). Preliminary studies show that chiropractic adjustments may be beneficial in autism (Alcantara et al. 2011). One case study showed resolution of cyclic vomiting after chiropractic care (Hubbard and Crisp 2010). From a review study in 2008, there was limited quality evidence for the use of SMT for children with otitis media (Pohlman and Holton-Brown 2012). Although there may be some benefit, there is not enough evidence at this time to recommend chiropractics for treatment of infant colic (Aase and Blaakaer 2013). There is weak evidence for the use of chiropractics to treat enuresis (Huang et al. 2011).

Safety There is insufficient research evidence about adverse events related to chiropractic and children. Clinical studies and systematic reviews from adult patients undergoing manual therapy report that mild to moderate adverse events are common and self-limiting, but serious adverse events are rare. Serious adverse events in chiropractic are much less common than for medications regularly prescribed for the same medical problems. More high-quality research specifically addressing adverse events and pediatric manual therapy is needed (Humphreys 2010).

Education In 2005, the World Health Organization published guidelines for the education of chiropractors (WHO 2005). In the United States, Canada, and many European countries, chiropractic is legally recognized and formal university degrees have been established. In these countries, the profession is regulated, and the prescribed educational qualifications are generally consistent.

Licensing of Practitioners Graduates of chiropractic schools receive the degree *Doctor of Chiropractic* (DC), and are eligible to seek licensure in all jurisdictions. The Council on Chiropractic Education (CCE) sets minimum guidelines for the 18 chiropractic colleges in the US.

VII. Clinical Hypnosis

Background The American Society of Clinical Hypnosis (ASCH) defines hypnosis as "… a state of inner absorption, concentration and focused attention… . Because hypnosis allows people to use more of their potential, learning self-hypnosis is the ultimate act of self-control" (ASCH 2014). Hypnosis is often described as purposeful daydreaming. Historically, the practice of attaining a trance or trance-like state for religious reasons, medicinal healing, or cultural initiation rites is well documented. The use of hypnosis in pediatrics was pioneered by Drs Milton Erickson and Erik Wright in the late 1950s. The field was furthered in the 1960s by Dr Franz Baumann, who implemented clinical hypnosis as treatment for a variety of pediatric medical conditions (Culbert and Olness 2010, p. 270–271).

Basics Clinical hypnosis is often used as a treatment to lessen pain. In general, the affective component of pain is processed in the medial aspect of the thalamus and sent to the anterior cingulate gyrus. A study was conducted by Rainville et al. to understand how hypnosis works. Volunteers were asked to place their hand into hot water and a PET scan was performed. The same volunteers underwent hypnosis, and a PET scan was repeated. With hypnosis, there was less activation of the anterior cingulate cortex, the part of brain that involves feelings of emotional distress and can influence pain inhibition. With hypnosis, there was no decrease in activation of the somatosensory cortex. The interpretation was that the brain may continue to register pain sensation during hypnosis, but patients are able to shift the pain experience away from emotional distress (Rainville et al. 1997).

The beauty of hypnosis is in its simplicity through use of language. All true hypnosis is self-hypnosis, which allows the patient to become empowered. The provider serves as a coach or facilitator. Establishment of rapport with a patient is essential to the process of hypnosis. With children, appreciation of the developmental and cognitive stage of a patient is also crucial for a successful hypnosis encounter. Children and adolescents experience *altered* mental states throughout the day when absorbed in video games, sports, watching movies, or reading exciting books. Referring to these feelings can bring a sense of familiarity and ease to the process of hypnosis. Complete absorption into the hypnosis enhances suggestibility, which is how a practitioner introduces therapeutic suggestions to reach goals for therapy. Formally, hypnosis has six stages: introduction, induction, intensification, therapeutic suggestion, re-alerting, and debriefing. Hypnosis in the younger pediatric patient is *fluid* or without strict attention to stages. Younger patients may be relatively active during the session. Induction may be achieved in a variety of ways dependent upon the developmental and cognitive level of the patient. Induction with young children may involve rocking, stroking, massaging, singing, playing with dolls or superheroes, or using items like pop-up books, pinwheels, or bubbles. Older children and adolescents may use favorite-place imagery, adventure imagery, magic carpet ride thoughts, abdominal breathing, helium balloon thoughts, imagery of a bucket of sand, or eye fixation. There may be physical signs during hypnosis indicating an *altered* mental state, such as fluttering of closed eyelids, slackening of facial muscles, head lowering, slowing and deepening of respirations, muscle twitching, and eye tearing. Children under the age of 10 years may not close their eyes during hypnosis. During hypnosis, patients are aware of their surroundings and may speak or signal with their hands. Of note, hypnosis susceptibility scales have not been accurate in predicting the success of hypnosis in children (Culbert and Olness 2010, p. 273).

Evidence The overwhelming evidence demonstrates hypnosis to be effective in many pediatric conditions including reduction of pain and anxiety. However, there are many criticisms of hypnosis studies including small sample sizes, flaws in methodology, and the idea that patients are not just undergoing hypnosis but undergoing relaxation or guided imagery. In addition, hypnosis is based on the *active participation* of the patient, and therefore double-blind studies are impossible. *Pain* is influenced by a person's developmental stage, prior experiences with pain, anxiety, physical and emotional stressors, and innate temperament. Hypnosis has been well-studied in adults with acute, chronic, and recurrent pain for many years. These techniques have virtually no side-effects and promote self-control. Self-hypnosis and imagery are routinely used to decrease pain and anxiety from painful procedures.

These modalities have become mainstream in many pediatric oncology centers. Studies have also noted that self-hypnosis can lessen nausea and vomiting (Senser and Kelly 2007). Extensive randomized controlled trials published by Uman et al. have concluded that hypnosis may alleviate pain and anxiety in needle-related procedures (Uman et al. 2013).

Studies have favored the use of hypnosis in treating behavioral conditions such as trichotillomania, enuresis, and thumb sucking (Saadat and Kain 2007). Hypnosis has also been studied in patients with functional respiratory conditions including dyspnea, hyperventilation, habit cough, throat clearing, and vocal cord dysfunction (Anbar 2012, p. 3). Dr Ran Anbar at Upstate Medical University (SUNY) has utilized hypnosis in the affiliated pediatric pulmonary center. Hypnosis research data from this center has included studies on functional chronic dyspnea (which improved in 19 % and completely resolved in 81 % of patients) and on habit cough (which resolved symptoms in 90 % of these cases) (Anbar 2012, pp. 229–230).

Safety Hypnosis is considered safe when implemented by a skilled practitioner. A full medical evaluation should be obtained prior to the use of hypnosis when treating pain, anxiety, and functional respiratory disorders to assess for underlying cause for symptoms. Hypnosis should never be used for purposes of entertainment.

Education Three of the large teaching organizations for clinical hypnosis include the American Society of Clinical Hypnosis (ASCH), National Pediatric Hypnosis Training Institute (NPHTI), and the New England Society of Clinical Hypnosis.

Licensure of Practitioners The ASCH has a certification program including requirements for beginner, intermediate, and advanced levels of training for licensed healthcare workers. Successful completion provides certification of basic training in hypnosis or certification as an approved consultant (www.asch.net). The NPHTI provides beginner, intermediate, and advanced training in pediatric hypnosis. The American Boards of Clinical Hypnosis include: American Board of Medical Hypnosis, American Board of Psychological Hypnosis, American Board of Hypnosis in Clinical Social Work, and the American Board of Dental Hypnosis. The American Board of Hypnosis in Nursing is being developed.

VIII. Healing Touch

Background Healing Touch (HT) therapy was developed in the 1980s by holistic nurse Janet Mentgen, RN. In 1989, Ms Mentgen formally created HT as an energy medicine program. In 1993, HT was certified by the American Holistic Nurses Association (AHNA). That same year, Ms. Mentgen formed The Colorado Center for Healing Touch, dedicated to bringing Healing Touch to millions of people throughout the world (Healing Touch Program 2013). HT believes that individuals possess energy fields and there also exists a universal energy field. Disruption of the energy system creates disease. HT provides relaxation through gentle touch to provide balance of mind, body, and spirit (Culbert and Olness 2010).

Basics The focus of HT is to assist in healing for the *highest good*. Typical sessions last up to one hour. The patient is fully clothed and lying or sitting in a comfortable position. The practitioner "centers" herself/himself and performs a body scan with her/his hands to detect subtle energy imbalances. After imbalances are assessed and treated, the practitioner re-alerts the patient to a fully alert state. The practitioner then re-evaluates the energy system, reviews symptoms, and discusses a follow-up self-care plan (Culbert and Olness 2010).

Evidence Research in HT is limited due to the lack of randomized controlled trials and the inability to elucidate a mechanism of action. There have been studies to suggest that HT may improve overall well-being. The pediatric literature on HT is sparse; however, HT is widely used in pediatric hospitals as an adjunctive therapy to reduce anxiety, pain, and stress (Culbert and Olness 2010). A pilot study was conducted to determine the effectiveness of HT on anxiety, stress, pain, pain medication usage, and selected physiological measures of hospitalized adults with sickle cell disease experiencing a vaso-occlusive pain episode. The sample size was small but there was some clinically significant benefit of HT on days 2–4 of the therapy (Thomas et al. 2013). Kemper et al. performed a pilot study with 9 pediatric cancer patients. The patients either received a 40-min rest session or a 20-min HT session within a 40-min rest session. Patients reported less stress, improved mood, and had lower heart rate variability compared with the same patient cohort who had 40 min of rest alone (Kemper et al. 2009) (Langler and Mansky 2012). A recent study in pediatric patients also demonstrated the feasibility of using energy therapy in the pediatric oncology patient population. In the study, the HT group showed significant decreases in scores for pain, stress, and fatigue for participants, parents, and caregivers. Furthermore, parents' perception of their children's pain decreased significantly for the HT group when compared with the group receiving reading/play activity (Wong et al. 2013).

Safety HT is generally considered safe when performed by trained professionals. There is no known risk in adding healing touch to conventional medical treatment.

Education Healing Touch Program (HTP) is an educational program that offers classes in HT as well as providing support for HT students, practitioners, and instructors.

Licensing of Practitioners In 1993, HT was certified by the AHNA. In 1996, Healing Touch International, Inc. was founded, and its purpose is to administer the HT certification process for practitioners and instructors. In 2008, the certification process was moved to the Healing Touch Certification Board.

IX. Supplements and Herbs

According to the CDC's National Center for Health Statistics surveys, the use of herbals and dietary supplements in the US has been increasing over the last 20 years. It is estimated that more than 50 % of US adults use at least one supplement

(Bailey et al. 2013). From a government study, an estimated 2.9 million children and adolescents used herbs or dietary supplements in 2007 and Americans spent over $30 billion on dietary supplements in that year (Nahin et al. 2009). Unfortunately, little is substantiated regarding the efficacy, purity, and at times safety of herbals and dietary supplements. Gardiner et al. noted that 72% adults who were using herbs were also taking other prescription medications and 84% were also taking over-the-counter medications (Gardiner et al. 2007).

The Oxford dictionary defines an herb as any plant with leaves, seeds, or flowers used for flavoring, food, medicine, or perfume. Herbal products that are designed for use in maintaining or improving health are known as phytomedicines. People around the world have used herbs to address a multitude of health issues for centuries. Analyses of archeological sites show that herbs were used long before the beginning of recorded history. The basis of medicinal properties of certain plants and their components has been the foundation for modern pharmacology. Individualized botanical treatments continue to be integral to the treatment plan of whole medical systems such as Ayurveda, Traditional Chinese Medicine, and Native American Medicine. According to the World Health Organization, 80% of the world's population still relies on herbal medicine as its primary form of healthcare. Germany and Canada consider herbs and supplements to be similar to medications. The European Union requires a premarket government approval for herbal products (Budzynska et al. 2012). This type of regulation is also mandated in Canada, where herbal products require preapproval evaluation through Natural Health Products (Health Canada 2012). In the US, the FDA considers herbals and dietary supplements as food products. Therefore, the degree of regulation is less stringent than that for prescription and over-the-counter medications. According to the Dietary Supplement Health and Education Act of 1994, "A supplemental product is intended to *supplement* the diet. It must contain at least one of the following ingredients (including vitamins; minerals; herbs or other botanicals; amino acids; and other substances) or their constituents. The product is intended to be taken orally as a pill, capsule, tablet or liquid; and the product information must be labeled on the front panel as being a dietary supplement" (NIH 2014).

It is the responsibility of the manufacturer to insure that a supplement or herbal product is pure and considered safe. All constituent products must be clearly documented on the label. Manufacturers are not obligated to report adverse events to the FDA, and substances that were on the market before 1994 are exempt from regulation. This is in contrast to prescription drugs and over-the-counter medications, for which manufacturers must provide safety and efficacy information to the FDA *before* the product reaches the market. If a product maintains a claim regarding *therapeutic efficacy*, there must be data provided for its support. Otherwise, supplements and herbs must have the following statement: "This statement has not been evaluated by the U.S. Food and Drug Administration (FDA). This product is not intended to diagnose, treat, cure, or prevent any disease."

Since 2007, new regulations have been created through the current Good Manufacturing Practices (cGMP). This includes verification that supplements and herbal products are processed, labeled, and packaged in compliance with standards. Thus, consumers should look for *GMP* on product labels. The Consumerlab seal implies documentation of the product's purity, potency, ingredients, and bioavailability, but it does not stipulate efficacy (Consumerlab 2013). The Federal Trade Commission requires that advertising of a product has foundational merit. The FDA may evaluate the safety of a product by conducting research on the product and tracking adverse side effects. Safety concerns can be cited through the FDA's voluntary MedWatch Program. It is the responsibility of all practitioners to report any adverse events noted from herbals and supplements. It is important to be mindful that *natural* does not necessarily mean *safe*. There was a lag of many years before ephedra was taken off the market despite reported safety concerns.

In our US system, the knowledgeable practitioner must communicate information to patients. Consumers believe that they are buying safe, *pure* herbal and supplement products. Yet, this may not be the case. Product authenticity may be compromised. A study by Miller et al. found that 10 % of random Chinese herbals purchased in New York City's Chinatown were adulterated (Miller 2007). Saper et al. discovered that 20 % of US and Indian Ayurdevic products purchased on the Internet contained lead, mercury, and/or arsenic that exceeded acceptable levels. In addition, of the products that contained mercury, 75 % were marked as GMP compliant (Saper et al. 2008).

According to NCCAM, biologically based practices are the most frequently used form of complementary therapy, and use of multivitamins is the most common. Up to 41 % of children take multivitamins. A study by Zhang et al. cited data from the Infant Feeding Practices Study II, a longitudinal survey conducted through the FDA and the CDC, which showed that 9 % of infants were given dietary botanical supplements or teas during their first year of life. Maternal herbal use, Hispanic ethnicity, and longer breast feeding were predictors for herb use in infants. The most common reasons for botanical use in infants were fussiness, colic, and relaxation (Zhang et al. 2011). According to the AAP Task Force on Complementary and Alternative Medicine, of teenagers who reported using CAM, almost 73 % used supplements and/or herbs (Kemper et al. 2008).

It is important to note that there may be great variation in herbal sources. Geographic location, time of plant harvest, and plant processing may influence potency of an herb. A study by Tachjian et al. revealed that more than 40 % of all herbal products failed to include the specified quantity of active ingredients on their label. There was concern regarding heavy metal contamination and intentional or unintentional pharmaceutical adulteration, including antibiotics, hormones, and nonsteroidal drugs. There was concern regarding prohibited animal and plant ingredients found in some herbal products. The study authors noted that in 2007, the FDA issued 9 safety alerts warning consumers to stop using 13 brands marketed as dietary supplements because testing revealed that the supplements contained undocumented prescription medication (Tachjian et al. 2010). Supplements may interact with medications and pose risks for medical procedures. It is crucial that health care providers ask questions regarding the use of over-the-counter supplements and herbals in a non-judgmental manner. Of note, St John's wort is a popular herb in the US used to treat mild to moderate depression, anxiety, and sleep disorders. This herb induces the hepatic cytochrome p450 pathway, which is involved in the metabolism of over 50 % of all prescription drugs. Therefore, there is potential for adverse effects such as hypertension and arrhythmias, and there is concern for decreased efficacy of certain antibiotics, immunosuppressants, chemotherapeutics, and psychotropic medications. St John's wort decreases prothrombin time, and Ginkgo biloba may increase risk of bleeding when used with anticoagulant or antiplatelet therapy. The active ingredient in garlic inhibits collagen-induced platelet aggregation. It is recommended that patients stop garlic supplements at least 10 days prior to surgery. Grapefruit juice also induces the cytochrome p450 pathway and should be used with caution in patients taking medications that utilize the CYP3A4 system for drug metabolism (Tachjian et al. 2010).

Reliable Sources National Center for Complementary and Alternative Medicine: http://www.nccam.nih.gov
NIH Office of Dietary Supplements: http://ods.od.nih.gov/HealthInformation/DS
U.S. FDA: http://www.fda.gov/Food/DietarySupplements
Natural Medicines Comprehensive Database: http://www.naturaldatabase.com
ConsumerLabs: http://www.consumerlabs.com
Natural Standard: http://www.naturalstandard.com
MedLinePlus: http://www.nlm.nih.gov/medlineplus/druginformation.com
MD Anderson Cancer Center: http://www.mdanderson.org/departments/CIMER
Memorial Sloan-Kettering Cancer Center: http://mskcc.org/mskcc/html/11570.cfm
Reference Book: The American Botanical Council (ABC) Clinical Guide to Herbs

Common Herbals and Supplements in Pediatrics: Echinacea

According to the 2007 National Health Interview Survey, the most common complementary health practice for children was use of natural products and the most common of these was Echinacea (Barnes et al. 2008a, b). Echinacea, or Purple Coneflower, has nine species. It is a member of the Compositae family, which includes asters, daisies, and sunflowers indigenous to North America. This plant has been used for hundreds of years for its healing effects. Native Americans of the Great Plains used it to heal wounds and introduced it to European settlers. Its use continued until the advent of antibiotics in the twentieth century. The three species primarily used for medicinal purposes are Echinacea angustifolia, Echinacea pallid, and Echinacea purpurea (Kemper 1996). The plant's ability as an immune stimulator is unclear. However, research suggests it may involve upregulation of tumor necrosis factor (Shah et al. 2007). Echinacea has also been found to modulate IgG responses, T cells phagocytosis, and cytokines (Kligler and Lee 2004).

On average, children suffer from 6 to 10 colds per year. There have been conflicting results regarding the efficacy of Echinacea on the course and/or prevention of upper respiratory infections. Unfortunately, there is a lack of uniformity as studies vary in Echinacea species, dosages, and frequencies of administration. Different parts of the plant are used therapeutically such as the flower, root, and/or stem. The potency of the active plant compounds can also vary with where, when, and how the plant was collected, processed, and stored. In 2002, Consumerlab reported that only 4 of the 11 brands of Echinacea tested contained the ingredients written on the label. Furthermore, approximately 10% did not contain Echinacea (Consumerlab

2013). In a 2005 Cochrane analysis including adult and pediatric studies, prevention with the use of Echinacea and treatment trials including placebo showed mixed results. In one randomized controlled study, a combination of Echinacea, vitamin C, and Propolis (a natural resinous product which is collected by honeybees) showed promise in the prevention of upper respiratory illness in children 1–5 years old. The total number of ill days and duration of illness were lower in the herbal preparation group (Cohen et al. 2004).

Madaus AG, or Echinacin, is the brand of Echinacea most studied in Germany. Branded as Echinaguard in the US by Nature's Way, it is made from pressed juice of Echinacea purpurea. The German Commission E approved 900 mg/day of Echinacea purpurea for the treatment of upper respiratory infections. A meta-analysis of 16 trials showed benefit of Echinacea for treatment but not prophylaxis of upper respiratory infection (Linde et al. 2006). In 2007, Shah et al. suggested added benefit for prophylaxis; however, they commented that large-scale randomized prospective studies are needed before delegating Echinacea as standard therapy for upper respiratory infections. They also stipulated the need for Echinacea standards including species, preparation, dose, and study objectives within the larger study parameters (Shah et al. 2007).

Echinacea is considered safe, at least for short-term use. The major side effects include gastrointestinal and skin reactions. Echinacea is a human cytochrome P450 3A4 enzyme inhibitor; therefore, there is potential that medications metabolized through cytochrome P450 1A2 may interact with Echinacea. Patients allergic to daisies, ragweed, chrysanthemums, and marigolds should be cautioned, as they may also be allergic to Echinacea. Patients with autoimmune disorders may react adversely to Echinacea. An interesting adult study with 713 patients with new-onset upper respiratory infection was performed in 2011. It showed that in patients who believed in the benefit of Echinacea and received pills, their illness was of shorter duration and less severe regardless of whether the pills they were given truly contained Echinacea (Barrett et al. 2011).

Dr Tieraona Low Dog of the University of Arizona states that there is sufficient data to suggest that Echinacea be started at the first indication of a cold. Echinacea tincture may be helpful in adequate doses, but the taste may need to be masked or improved with natural flavorings like cherry. Her recommended dose: Echinacea glycerites 3 mL for children 5–12 years old every 4–6 h for the first 2–3 days. For children 13 and older, she recommends twice that dose. In addition, she suggests that it is best to reassure parents and patients that symptomatic treatment is best for routine upper respiratory infections and *no treatment* may be the best treatment (Low Dog 2008).

Common Herbals and Supplements in Pediatrics: Chamomile

Chamomile is one of the oldest medicinal herbs. It is a member of the Compositae family and has 2 common varieties known as German chamomile (*Chamomilla recutita*) and Roman chamomile (*Chamaemelum nobile*). Most research has been with German chamomile. An herb used commonly by Hispanic patients, chamomile is known in Spanish as *manzanilla*. It is typically used for skin rashes, colic, as a mild sedative, and for diarrhea. The medicinal ingredients of the dried flowers are extracted with water, ethanol, or methanol. Chamomile extract usually contains 50% ethanol. The dried flowers of chamomile contain flavonoids and terpenoids, the medicinal properties of which are thought to be effective, but their exact mechanisms of action are still unknown. Chamazulene is an antioxidant that inhibits leukotriene B4 and may be responsible for chamomile's potential anti-inflammatory properties (Safayhi et al. 1994). The flowers also contain flavonoids such as apigenin (Srivastava et al. 2010). It is thought that the flavonoid component may have an anxiolytic effect by either affecting gamma butyric acid (GABA), noradrenalin (NA), dopamine (DA), and serotonin transmission or by influencing the hypothalamic pituitary adrenocortical axis. Apigen has been found to bind to benzodiazepine receptors and decrease GABA-induced activity (Amsterdam et al. 2009).

Chamomile tea is enjoyed by millions of people every day. The tea contains flower powder either in pure form or combined with other herbs. The whole chamomile plant is used in herbal beers and lotions to improve pain and reduce inflammation. The vaporized essential oils, from the dried flowers, are used in aromatherapy for relaxation.

Two clinical trials have studied the effects of chamomile in patients with colic. One was a prospective, randomized, double-blind, placebo-controlled study. Sixty-eight healthy newborns (ages 2–8 weeks) with colic were given either placebo or herbal tea consisting of German chamomile, licorice, vervain, fennel, and balm mint. The colic episodes were treated with up to 150 mL per dose up to a maximum of 3 doses per day. At the end of 1 week, a parental survey showed 57% elimination of colic with tea versus 26% with placebo ($p < 0.01$). A related randomized, double- blind, placebo-controlled trial studied 93 colicky breast-fed infants. The infants were randomized to placebo or standardized German chamomile extract, fennel, and lemon balm twice daily for 1 week. The crying time decreased in 85.4% of the treated group versus 48.9% in the placebo group ($p < 0.005$). No adverse effects were observed in either study (Gardiner 2007). The use of apple pectin-chamomile extract in 39 of 79 children with acute noncomplicated diarrhea showed improvement in diarrhea sooner in the treated group (85%) versus placebo (58%). A multicenter followup randomized, double-blind, placebo-controlled study by Becker et al. of 255 patients ages 6 months to 6 years showed superior symptom resolution of diarrhea in the treated group (Becker et al. 2006).

Chamomile is regarded as a sleep aid and mild tranquilizer. It is known that apigenin binds to benzodiazepine receptors in the brain. However, there are few studies to confirm these clinical attributes. Zick et al. performed a randomized, double-blind, placebo-controlled pilot study of 34 adult patients with DSM-IV diagnosed primary insomnia. The study showed that chamomile may benefit daytime functioning and there were no differences in side effects between the groups (Zick et al. 2011). Anxiety disorders are common mental health conditions in adults. In childhood the incidence of anxiety disorders is estimated at 8%. There are several types of anxiety disorders including generalized anxiety disorder (GAD), panic disorder, separation anxiety disorder, and phobic disorder. GAD may manifest physical and psychological limitations. The conventional treatment is with benzodiazepines, but these medications may be associated with untoward side effects. Selective serotonin reuptake inhibitor antidepressants are also used for GAD, but they may also produce side effects. German chamomile has traditionally been used for relaxation and use is supported by animal studies. A study by Amsterdam et al. studied 57 adult patients with DSM-IV axis I diagnosis of GAD. German chamomile in 220 mg capsules or placebo was initiated at 1 capsule for week 1 and increased to 2 capsules for week 2. Some were increased to a maximum of 5 capsules daily through weeks 5 through 8. The study showed that chamomile may have modest anxiolytic activity in patients with mild to moderate GAD (Amsterdam et al. 2009).

Studies have suggested that chamomile may be helpful in wound healing, atopic dermatitis, weeping skin conditions, and decubitus ulcers. These studies had limitations and need to be validated on a larger scale before implementing routine use of chamomile in dermatologic conditions (Gardiner 2007).

It is possible that people who are sensitive to other members of the Compositae family such as ragweed may be at risk for allergic-type reactions to chamomile. There have been cases of interaction with cyclosporine in patients who were post-renal transplant. This is believed to be secondary to inhibition of P450 CYP 1A2 and 3A4. Potential interactions may also exist with warfarin, also due to chamomile's effects on the P450 system (Gardiner 2007).

Common Herbals and Supplements in Pediatrics: Peppermint

Peppermint, or *Mentha piperita,* is a perennial member of the mint family that grows in Europe and North America. The peppermint oil is extracted from stem, leaves, and flowers. It has been used for centuries as a digestive aid and has more recently been used to alleviate symptoms of irritable bowel disease, non-ulcer dyspepsia, and tension headaches. Menthol is the primary essential oil and the active ingredient of peppermint (Kligler and Chaudhary 2007). Menthol is a cyclic monoterpene that is used to help alleviate muscle aches and respiratory congestion. The most common side effects of peppermint include allergic reactions, esophageal pain, heartburn, and rectal burning (Chiou and Nurko 2010). Peppermint oil has been found to relax the tone of the lower esophageal sphincter and therefore has potential for aggravating gastroesophageal reflux. Enteric-coated preparations of peppermint oil are typically used (Charrois et al. 2006). Peppermint has been shown, in a few studies, to decrease colonic spasms during barium enema and colonoscopy examinations in adults (Kline et al. 2001).

Research on the possible benefit of peppermint has focused on gastrointestinal conditions, primarily functional gastrointestinal disorders. Irritable bowel syndrome (IBS) is the most commonly diagnosed gastrointestinal disorder in the developed world. Estimated adult prevalence is 5–25 %. The treatment of IBS remains challenging as there is no gold standard for long-term treatment. Studies in adult patients with IBS have shown potential promise with peppermint oil. However, there have been limitations to interpretation due to the significant heterogeneity of patient populations, who may have conditions such as lactose intolerance, bacterial overgrowth of small intestine, or celiac disease. Ford et al. performed a systematic review and meta-analysis that showed that fiber, antispasmodics, and peppermint oil were all more effective than placebo in the treatment of irritable bowel syndrome (Ford and Talley 2008). Capello et al. performed a prospective double-blind placebo-controlled randomized trial involving 50 adult patients with IBS. The treatment group was given 2 enteric peppermint capsules twice daily for 4 weeks, which resulted in a daily peppermint dose of 900 mg. The evaluation of symptoms at 4 weeks showed that 75% of patients treated with peppermint oil had at least a 50% reduction of the basal symptom score ($p < 0.009$) and this was also statistically significant at 8 weeks (Capello et al. 2007).

Functional abdominal pain and IBS are commonly seen in pediatric practices. Prevalence estimates are variable, but community and school-based studies estimate the prevalence of weekly abdominal pain to be 13–38%. It is estimated that 24% of children may have abdominal pain that persists more than 8 weeks (Hyams et al. 1996). Abdominal pain is associated with poorer quality of life, psychological co-morbidities, school absenteeism, and parental work absences (Saps et al. 2009). Kline studied 42 children with IBS in a randomized double-blind controlled study. Peppermint oil 0.1 mL (1 capsule enteric coated) was prescribed 3 times daily if the child weighed 30–45 kg, and 2 capsules were prescribed 3 times daily if the child weighed more than 45 kg. The placebo used was arachis oil. Pre- and post-study measures at day 1 and 14 were recorded. Seventy-six percent of patients in the peppermint group reported improvement in symptom severity at day 14. This was in contrast to 19% in the control group ($p < 0.001$). The mean severity in pain was less in the peppermint group ($p < 0.03$). There were no adverse effects described in this study (Kline et al. 2001).

Common Herbals and Supplements in Pediatrics: St. John's Wort

St John's wort (*Hypericum perforatum*) is a commonly used herb in the US. Its preparations are extracted from the plant's leaves and flowers, which are harvested either before or immediately after the plant flowers. Hypericin and hyperforin are among at least 10 active ingredients found in St John's wort. Although the exact mechanism is unknown, it is believed that these two products bind the neuroreceptors and inhibit the re-uptake of serotonin, norepinephrine, and dopamine (Culbert and Olness 2010). It has been demonstrated that hypericum decreases the expression of the serotonin receptor itself (Kasper et al. 2006). Historically, St. John's wort has been used for treatment of insect bites, burns, and wounds as a balm. In the scientific literature, its potential use in treating depression was initially described by Josey and Tackett (Josey and Tackett 1999). In a study involving children and adolescents at a primary care clinic, more than 50% of patients who reported taking herbal medications were using hypericum (Soh and Walter 2008).

Due to many factors, there may be variations in the chemical constituents of a St. John's wort plant. Therefore, the herbal products may vary in potency and purity. There have been reports of St. John's wort products sold in the United States with contents different from what was stated on the label. There have also been reported cases of contamination with cadmium in some products. Most product labels claim 0.3 % hypericin, but this may vary from product to product (Charrois et al. 2007). Of note, St. John's wort should be stored in an opaque container due to possible interaction of light with plant constituents (Kemper 2010). St. John's wort has been studied extensively in Europe for more than 20 years. Kasper et al. studied 332 adult patients with mild to moderate depression who were randomized to either placebo or St. John's wort WS 5570. St. John's wort was shown to be significantly more effective than placebo with at least similar efficacy and better tolerability compared to standard antidepressant drugs. The dosing schedules utilized were found to be safe and well tolerated (Kasper et al. 2010). A related study by Szegedi et al. compared hypericum extract WS 5570 to paroxetime in 251 adult patients with moderate to severe depression in a randomized double-blind multicenter trial using the Hamilton depression scale as the primary outcome. Patients were treated with hypericum or paroxetine daily. At the end of 6 weeks, Hamilton depression total score decreased 56.6 % in the hypericum group and 44.8 % in the paroxetine group. Adverse event incidence was 0.035 in the hypericum group and 0.060 in the paroxetine group. Szegedi et al. concluded that "in the treatment of moderate to severe major depression, hypericum extract WS 5570 is at least as effective as paroxetine and is better tolerated" (Szegedi et al. 2005). Studies from German-speaking countries seem favorable for its use in treating depression. A Cochrane review published in 2008 concluded that studies of hypericum extract revealed it to be superior to placebo in adult patients with major depression. There appears to be similar efficacy between St. John's wort and antidepressants (tricyclics, tetracyclics, and SSRIs). And overall, St. John's wort appears to have fewer side effects than conventional medications for this condition (Linde 2008).

Few studies have assessed the efficacy of St. John's wort in pediatrics, with no randomized, controlled trials to date. Most have had small sample sizes and have been open-label studies. Simeon et al. performed a prospective, open-label outpatient study of 26 patients ages 12–17 who had major depressive symptoms. Only 11 patients completed the 8-week study. Nine of the 11 patients showed significant clinical response as measured with Clinical Global Improvement scores (Simeon et al. 2005).

Hypericum is well tolerated. Adverse events are estimated at 1–3 % of all patients. The most common adverse effects include fatigue, headache, dry mouth, and stomach discomfort. There is a possibility of allergic skin reactions and photosensitivity. Pediatric studies have found tolerance up to 8 weeks, and the most common side effects in children include dizziness, diarrhea, and alterations in appetite. Drug interactions may be significant if a patient is taking a medication that is metabolized via CYP450 3A4 enzyme, like carbamazepine, cyclosporine, or protease inhibitors, concomitantly with St. John's wort. Importantly, increased metabolism of oral contraceptives may also occur. Warfarin metabolism may also be affected, resulting in an increased risk of thromboembolic events, and there is increased risk of serotonin syndrome with concomitant use of SSRI medications. To date, there is no *standard* dosing for hypericum. The pediatric dose range is from 300 to 900 mg/day in divided doses. The extracts are available in capsule, tablet, or caplet forms (Barnes et al. 2008a, b).

Common Herbals and Supplements in Pediatrics: Butterbur (Petasites hybridus)

Butterbur is a native European plant that has been used for centuries for its medicinal properties. The active ingredients are petasin and isopetasin. The petasins are extracted from the root of the plant and have an antispasmodic effect on smooth muscle and vascular walls. Petasins have been shown to inhibit the synthesis of leukotrienes, decrease mast cell priming, and thus decrease histamine concentrations (Culbert and Olness 2010). Petadolex, a commercial butterbur product produced in Germany, has been available in the United States as an herbal product since 1997. This product has been shown to be efficacious for migraine prophylaxis in adults. The 2012 Guidelines from the American Headache Society and the American Academy of Neurology consider butterbur as a level "A" medication for prevention of episodic migraine. This distinction is due to its efficacy in at least 2 high-quality randomized controlled trials. These guidelines were specific to studies involving patients at least 18 years of age (Loder et al. 2012). Pediatric data is accumulating. One open-label study involved 108 children, ages 6–17 years, who had a history of migraines per the International Headache Society classification. A Petadolex 25 mg capsule was given twice daily for 6- to 9-year-olds, and a 50 mg capsule was dosed twice daily for 10- to 17-year-old patients for a total of 4 months. Response was defined as at least 50 % reduction in monthly migraine attacks. Approximately 85.7 % of the younger children and 74.1 % of the older children responded to Petadolex treatment. Overall, Petadolex was well tolerated with a total of 8 adverse events, including 4 cases of mild belching or nausea and 1 case of moderate abdominal pain. These events did not result in withdrawal from the study (Pothmann and Danesch 2005).

Pediatric dosing of butterbur is 50–75 mg twice daily and is well tolerated. Side effects include mild eructation, nausea, abdominal discomfort, and flatulence. The adult literature estimates the side effect of eructation to be 20 % and other side effects of nausea and stomach discomfort to be much less common. All side effects from butterbur appear to be transient and mild. It is important that commercial products of butterbur are used and that the drug is free of pyrrolizidine alkaloid (PA) and labeled as such. There have been no reported allergic reactions to butterbur, but it is in the aster, daisy, and sunflower family, and so there is a theoretical risk of allergy in patients sensitive to those plants. There have been no known clinical drug interactions with butterbur. It is recommended that anticholinergics be avoided, as pyrrolizidine alkaloids use the CYP3A4 enzyme system for metabolism. Caution is suggested with concomitant use of CYP3A4 inducers (Sadler et al. 2007).

Common Herbals and Supplements in Pediatrics: Melatonin

Melatonin is a naturally occurring hormone primarily produced in the pineal gland but also in the gastrointestinal tract and retina. Melatonin acts on the MT1 and MT2 receptors in the suprachiasmatic nucleus of the hypothalamus and is intimately involved with the circadian rhythm (Kostoglou-Athanassiou 2013). The production of melatonin is enhanced by darkness and blocked by light. Melatonin levels are 10–30 times higher at night than during the day. The ability to produce melatonin can be affected if there is light exposure at night. Due to its influence on sleep-wake cycles, melatonin research has focused on specific groups (shift workers, travelers crossing multiple time zones, and patients within an intensive care unit setting) who may experience disruption of the normal melatonin production due to exposure to light during typical evening hours. Interestingly, melatonin levels may differ in patients with mood disorders, insomnia, and Alzheimer's disease. Changes in melatonin levels have also been noted in relation to aging (Kemper 2010). Melatonin is classified as a dietary supplement in the United States but as a natural health product by Health Canada. Several studies have suggested that melatonin may be beneficial for prevention and treatment of jet lag, but the evidence is not overwhelming. Cochrane reviews have shown that melatonin taken before sleep time at the destination area improves jet lag when persons travel through five or more time zones. Melatonin doses range from 0.5 to 5 mg (Kostoglou-Athanassiou 2013). Immediate-release preparations of melatonin are recommended for patients having difficulty falling asleep and sustained-release preparations can benefit those who cannot stay asleep (Kemper 1996).

It is estimated that sleep-wake disorders affect approximately 20 % of children and adolescents. This may negatively impact their quality of life (Suresh and Pianosi 2006). Also, acute and chronic medical conditions increase the potential for nonrestorative sleep (Lewandowski et al. 2011). In 2005, Buscemi et al. reviewed the literature for melatonin use in primary sleep disorders. Two double-blind randomized controlled studies included children ages 6–12 who suffered from chronic sleep-onset insomnia. They were randomized to either placebo or 5 mg of fast-release melatonin nightly for 4 weeks. The authors concluded that melatonin is not effective in treating most primary sleep disorders with short-term use, but improves sleep-onset latency by 16.7 min (Buscemi 2005). Promising results for the use of melatonin in children with secondary sleep disorders exist. A meta-analysis of three cross-over studies involving 66 children with developmental disabilities, Rett syndrome, and tuberous sclerosis showed a significant improvement of sleep-onset latency of 18 min (Shamseer and Vohra 2009). There has been considerable interest in studying melatonin for patients with attention-deficit/ hyperactivity disorder (ADHD). It is estimated that chronic sleep-onset insomnia may occur in up to 28 % of nonmedicated children with ADHD (Hoebert et al. 2009). Van der Heijden et al. investigated the potential effects of melatonin in children 6–12 years old with ADHD and chronic sleep-onset insomnia. The group conducted a randomized double-blind placebo-controlled trial of 105 patients who were given 3 or 6 mg of melatonin, depending on their weight, or they were given placebo once nightly for 4 weeks. Melatonin improved sleep onset significantly ($p < 0.001$). Total sleep time increased with melatonin versus placebo ($p = 0.01$). No changes in behavior, cognition, or quality of life were observed, and there were no significant adverse events. Hoebert et al. performed long-term followup with the previous patients through parental questionnaire. The response rate was 93 % and mean followup was 3.7 years. The study reported that 65 % of children were still using melatonin nightly, and discontinuation of melatonin resulted in adverse sleep onset time in 92 % of patients. Interestingly, improvement in behavior was described in 71 % of patients. Three children discontinued melatonin due to side effects of dizziness, headache, abdominal pain, visual disturbance, excessive daytime sedation, and perspiration, but all side effects resolved once melatonin was discontinued. There were no serious adverse events (Hoebert et al. 2009). It has been reported that melatonin causes abnormal physiological changes in some patients with autism spectrum disorders (ASDs). These include abnormal circadian patterns, lower mean melatonin concentrations, and lower levels of urinary melatonin metabolites. A recent study demonstrated a higher level of polymorphisms in the ASMT gene, which is involved in melatonin synthesis. This was noted in 250 patients with ASDs versus control patients ($p = 0.0006$). These polymorphisms were associated with decreased blood melatonin levels ($p < 0.00001$). Melatonin was given a grade of "A" by the author, which implied its use being supported by at least 2 prospective randomized controlled trials or 1 systematic review (Rossignol 2009).

The typical dose of melatonin for sleep disturbance is 1–5 mg given 30–60 min before bed. The safety of long-term use of melatonin has not been evaluated. Although recent studies have not revealed significant side effects from melatonin use, it should be supervised by a healthcare professional. There have been concerns regarding possible effects of melatonin on luteinizing hormone. Also, a study published in Lancet in 1998 described an increase in seizure activity when melatonin was given to 6 children with seizure disorder (Sheldon 1998). This finding has not been duplicated in subsequent research reports. Caution is recommended in patients with autoimmune disorders due to melatonin's possible effect on the immune system. Caution is also advised with concomitant use of antihypertensive medication, especially extended-release nifedipine (DerMarderosian 1996).

Common Herbals and Supplements in Pediatrics: Curcumin

Tumeric is a spice derived from the rhizomes of *Curcuma longa*, a member of the ginger family. The yellow color of turmeric comes from curcuminoids. Curcumin is the primary cuminoid in turmeric. Tumeric has a long history of medicinal use in India. Its anti-inflammatory properties have been recognized for centuries. In India, the average intake of turmeric for a 60 kg person is 2–2.5 g/day, resulting in curcumin intake of approximately 60–100 mg daily. It appears that humans can tolerate increased doses of curcumin without significant side effects (Suskind et al. 2013).

It has been well-established that most chronic illnesses are caused by dysregulated inflammation and, therefore, therapy aimed at decreasing abnormal inflammation may be therapeutic. Curcumin has been found to interfere with numerous cytokines, protein kinases, transcription factors, adhesion molecules, and enzymes that are instrumental in the inflammatory process (Aggarwal and Harikumar 2009). Hanai et al. studied 89 adult patients with ulcerative colitis in remission with a randomized double-blind mulitcenter trial on the possible effect of curcumin in maintaining ulcerative colitis disease quiescence. All patients received either sulfasalazine or mesalamine. Forty-five patients received 1 g of curcumin twice daily and 44 patients received placebo for 6 months. The clinical activity index (CIA) and endoscopic index (EI) were obtained at baseline. The clinical index was determined every 2 months, at the end of the study, and 6 months thereafter. Only 2 patients (4.65%) in the curcumin group relapsed during the 6-month study, compared with 20.5% in the placebo group ($p=0.04$). Curcumin improved the CIA ($p=0.038$) and the EI ($p=0.0001$) (Hanai et al. 2006).

Studies of curcumin in pediatrics are limited. Suskind et al. studied curcumin tolerability in a prospective study with 11 pediatric patients whose inflammatory bowel disease was either quiescent or mild. Six of the patients had Crohn's disease and 5 had ulcerative colitis. Six patients were taking mesalamine and 5 patients were under antitumor necrosis factor therapy. Maintenance medications were continued during the study. Patients were given 500 mg of curcumin twice daily for 3 weeks, which was titrated up to a final dose of 2 g twice daily by week 6 for 3 weeks. Nine patients finished the study. Three patients had improvement in validated measures known as the Pediatric Crohn's Disease Activity Index and the Pediatric Ulcerative Colitis Activity Index. Two patients with ulcerative colitis had decreased scores, indicating remission. The patients tolerated the curcumin well (Suskind et al. 2013).

Curcumin appears to be well-tolerated although specific dosing has yet to be determined. Further studies need to be performed regarding safety, tolerability, and efficacy of curcumin in pediatrics. There are no standard dosages of curcumin for children. Curcumin may affect blood clotting, and thus caution is recommended with medications that alter this process.

Common Herbals and Supplements in Pediatrics: Prebiotics and Probiotics

Prebiotics are defined as nondigestible food ingredients that may favorably affect growth and/or activity of at least one probiotic bacteria. In contrast, probiotics are defined as oral supplements or food products that contain a specified number of viable microorganisms capable of altering host microflora in order to have potential health benefits. The probiotics most studied include Lactobacillus rhamnosus GG, Bifidobacterium lactis, and Streptococcus thermophilicus. It is hypothesized that probiotics can predominate over potential pathogenic microorganisms in the gastrointestinal tract through production of small molecular products. In turn, these products may have immune modulating capacities. A significant amount of research in the use of probiotics for multiple health conditions has been published in the adult and pediatric literature. There are fluctuations in policy recommendations due to ongoing research. The use of individual probiotic products, or combinations thereof, may be difficult to recommend, given the diversity of probiotic strains, number of organisms, dose fluctuations, and duration of treatment. Furthermore, there may be diversity within the products themselves. A Consumerlab report posted 11/23/13 found that 30% of probiotic supplements did not contain the listed amounts of organism stated on the label. Of the 19 probiotics sold for humans, 5 contained only 16–56% of the listed organisms. Tod Cooperman, MD, President of Consumerlab, expressed concern over some companies' inclusion of a footnote stating that the number of organisms was counted *at the time of manufacture*. He emphasized that individual probiotic products need to comply with their label at the time of purchase. Probiotics are sensitive to their environment and may be altered by heat, humidity, and light, depending on the product. In addition, some products need to be refrigerated even before opening.

Probiotics are one of the fastest-growing dietary supplements in the United States. Nutrition Business Journal estimated that sales of probiotics increased by 24.5% in 2012 to a new high of $ 947 million. A Consumerlab survey in 2012 revealed that 37.4% women and 30.5% men were taking probiotics. Some probiotic products cost nearly $ 1 per dose (Consumerlab 2013).

Probiotics are used for a variety of conditions. Notably, promising results regarding the efficacy of probiotics in the treatment of acute infectious diarrhea have been reported in well-designed randomized controlled studies. Szymanski et al. conducted a randomized controlled double-blind placebo-controlled study demonstrating that LGG administration decreased the mean duration of acute rotavirus diarrhea by 40 h. This result was not observed with other causes of acute diarrhea. The study further demonstrated that LGG shortened the time needed for intravenous hydration by 18 h (Szymański et al. 2006).

Canani et al. studied the efficacy of five different probiotic preparations in the treatment of acute diarrhea in a prospective single-blind randomized controlled study involving 571 children ages 3 months to 3 years. Children were randomized to either oral rehydration alone; Lactobacillus rhamnosus (formerly Lactobacillus casei strain GG or Lactobacillus GG); S boulardii; Bacillus clausii; a mix of L delbrueckii var bulgaricus, Stretococcus thermophilus, L acidophilus, and Bifidobacterium bifidum; or E faecium strain SF68. The probiotic preparations were given orally for 5 days. Mean diarrheal duration for children who received L rhamnosus strain GG was 78.5 h. Those who received the mixed preparation had mean diarrhea duration of 70 versus 115 h in the oral rehydration group ($p < 0.001$). The number of daily stools decreased significantly 1 day after treatment in the L rhamnosus and in the mixed group versus control ($p < 0.001$). The authors concluded that the efficacy of probiotics in the treatment of acute diarrhea in this population was strain-dependent and that probiotics should be considered as and prescribed as medications (Canani et al. 2007).

A 2010 Cochrane review that examined probiotics in the treatment of acute infectious diarrhea found 63 studies and a total of 8014 patients. Fifty-six trials recruited infants and young children. The authors concluded that rehydration together with probiotic use was safe and beneficial, with shorter duration of diarrhea (overall by 25 h) and decreased stool frequency (Allen et al. 2010). Hempel et al. studied probiotic use in the prevention and treatment of antibiotic-associated diarrhea. There were 87 randomized controlled trials, of which 16 focused on children ages 0–17. The findings demonstrated that probiotic use reduced the risk of antibiotic-associated diarrhea ($p = 0.002$). The authors stated that although previous studies showed that efficacy may be strain-specific, this was not observed in their study. Furthermore, deciding which population may benefit from adjunctive use of probiotics has yet to be determined. There were no noted serious adverse effects from probiotic use. However, there have been rare cases of bacterial sepsis and fungemia linked to probiotic use (Hempel et al. 2012).

Another study area of probiotic use has been with inflammatory bowel disease (IBD). There are estimates that 40–70 % of adults and children with IBD use complementary therapies, including probiotics. A Cochrane review of probiotic use in adults with ulcerative colitis showed similar efficacy of probiotics when compared with standard anti-inflammatory medications. In addition, similar results were found with adults who had ileoanal pouchitis. The probiotic product most often used in these studies was VSL#3, which contains S thermophilus, Bifidobacterium species and Lactobacillus species (Thomas and Greer 2010). Miele et al. studied 29 newly diagnosed pediatric patients with ulcerative colitis randomized to either placebo or VSL#3, in addition to the standard steroid induction and mesalamine maintenance therapy. Thirteen patients (92.8 %) of the VSL#3-treated patients achieved remission versus 36.4 % ($p < 0.001$) of the patients receiving placebo. Furthermore, the relapse rate with VSL#3 was 21 % versus 73.3 % without VSL#3 within 1 year of followup. No clinical or biochemical adverse events were associated with VSL#3 use (Miele et al. 2009).

It is well documented that the newborn gut microflora is an integral constituent of the developing immune system. Preterm infants may be exposed to a variety of factors that may adversely affect the integrity of this defense system. It is theorized that probiotics may assist the preterm infant by protecting the gut microflora and its environment. Probiotics have been found to *upregulate* immunity and increase anti-inflammatory cytokines. Also, probiotics can impede the intestinal permeability of pathogens associated with the development of necrotizing enterocolitis (NEC). Deshpande et al. published results of a systematic review of 11 randomized, controlled trials involving 2176 infants less than 34 weeks gestation. Infants treated with probiotics had significantly reduced all-cause mortality and NEC ($p < 0.00001$) (Deshpande et al. 2010; Tarnow-Mordi et al. 2010). A recent Cochrane review included 16 trials with 2842 infants to assess the possible role of probiotics in preventing necrotizing enterocolitis with preterm infants. Preterm was defined as < 37 weeks gestation and/or weighing less than 2500 g. The review stated that probiotic use significantly reduced the occurrence of severe NEC (stage II or more) and mortality, but did not affect the incidence of nosocomial sepsis. Results for extremely low birth weight infants could not be interpreted. There were no systemic infections reported with probiotic administration. The authors advocated the implementation of probiotics for infants greater than 1000 g (Alfaleh 2011).

There have been concerns regarding the overall safety of probiotics, especially in patients who are immunocompromised, including sick preterm infants. In most instances of illness after probiotic use, the offending organism has been from the patient's own flora. Large studies including premature infants have not reported increased incidence of sepsis associated with the use of probiotics. Indeed, more research needs to be conducted in order to safely recommend particular probiotic products. At this time, probiotics need not be approved by the FDA. In the future, regulation will be important as probiotics are recommended for prevention and treatment of specific illnesses.

X. Homeopathy

Background Homeopathy is a system of alternative medicine developed in 1796 by Samuel Hahnemann in Germany. It is based on the doctrine of *like cures like*. The word "homeopathy" is derived from the Greek words homoios (similar) and pathos (suffering or disease). In the basic belief of homeopathy, a substance that causes the symptoms of a disease in a healthy person will cure similar symptoms in a sick person (Culbert and Olness 2009; Hahnemann 1833). A common example of use of homeopathy is that if a person suffers from runny nose and watery eyes, treatment could include a diluted dose of onion. According to the 2007 National Health Interview Survey, which included a comprehensive survey of the use of complementary health practices by Americans, an estimated 3.9 million adults and 910,000 children used homeopathy in the previous year (Nahin et al. 2009). Patients with chronic conditions often turn to homeopathy as they are dissatisfied with conventional treatments.

Basics The low concentration of substances in homeopathic remedies, which often lack even a single molecule of the diluted substance, has been the basis of questions about the effects of the remedies since the 19th century (Ernst 2005). Modern advocates of homeopathy have proposed a concept of *water memory*, in which water *remembers* the substances mixed in it, and transmits the effect of those substances when consumed. This concept is inconsistent with the current understanding of matter, and water memory has never been demonstrated to have any detectable effect, biological or otherwise (Teixeira 2007). Many people believe that the placebo effect leads to the success of homeopathy.

Homeopathy is used in children of all ages. In infants, substances like Chamomilla are used for teething. For colic, infants may benefit from Pulsatilla, Arsenicum, Nux vomica, and Sulphur. Homeopathic remedies are also used for asthma, allergies, eczema, attention deficit hyperactivity disorder (ADHD), and constipation. A wide variety of homeopathic remedies are now available at grocery stores, corner drug stores and on-line. As homeopathy should be individualized, self-medication may not always be effective. It is best practice to have patients consult with an experienced homeopath for best results.

Evidence A systematic review published in 2007 reviewed 327 articles to assess the evidence of any type of therapeutic or preventive intervention testing homeopathy for childhood and adolescent ailments. Altunc et al. concluded that "the evidence from rigorous clinical trials of any type of therapeutic or preventive intervention testing homeopathy for childhood and adolescent ailments is not convincing enough for recommendations in any condition" (Altunc et al. 2007). Since that review in 2007, some studies have demonstrated efficacy of homeopathy in certain conditions. A study of 230 children with acute otitis media (AOM) treated with homeopathy showed the resolution rate to be 2.4 times faster than in placebo controls. There were no complications observed in the study group, and compared to conventional treatment the approach was 14% cheaper (Frei and Thurneysen 2001a, pp. 180–182). A study from 2011 suggests that homeopathic ear drops are moderately effective in treating otalgia in children with AOM and may be most effective in the early period after a diagnosis of AOM (Taylor and Jacobs 2011).

Regarding ADHD, one study showed that in cases where treatment of a hyperactive child is not urgent, homeopathy is a valuable alternative to methylphenidate. In preschoolers, homeopathy appears a particularly useful treatment for ADHD (Frey and Thurneysen 2001b, pp. 183–188). Looking at asthma, a study of 30 asthmatic children provided evidence that homeopathic medicines as prescribed by experienced homeopathic practitioners reduce severity of asthma symptoms (Shafei et al. 2012). A study on atopic dermatitis confirmed a positive therapeutic effect of homeopathy in atopic children (Rossi et al. 2012). The results of a prospective, multicenter, observational study demonstrated the interest of homeopathic medicines for the prevention and treatment of migraine attacks in children. A significant decrease in the frequency, severity, and duration of migraine attacks was observed and, consequently, reduced absenteeism from school (Danno et al. 2013).

Safety Homeopathy is considered to be quite safe. The medical literature contains no reference to adverse effects of remedies diluted beyond 6C (dilution to 10^{-12}). There are isolated instances of adverse reactions to lower dilutions; however, these were likely due to substandard quality of care. Homeopathy may cause an initial aggravation of symptoms but this is generally regarded as a favorable early response and subsides over time. There is little oversight of homeopathic medications, so practitioners should take note of any adverse reactions and report them appropriately (Kuehn 2009). Homeopathic drug interactions have not been published so one can assume that they are rare, especially given the dilution of the medications.

Education In 1900, there were 22 homeopathic medical schools in the U.S. Although none of those schools presently exist, a growing number of schools and training programs have opened in recent years. Currently in the US, approximately 25 schools teach homeopathy.

Licensing According to the NCCAM, laws regulating the practice of homeopathy in the United States vary from state to state. Usually, individuals licensed to practice medicine or another health care profession can legally practice homeopathy. In some states, nonlicensed professionals may practice homeopathy. The National Board of Homeopathic Examiners is a multidisciplinary examining and certifying board for homeopathic professionals. Certification is also offered through the Council for Homeopathic Certification. Arizona, Connecticut, and Nevada are the only states with homeopathic licensing boards for doctors of medicine and osteopathic medicine. Some states explicitly include homeopathy within the scope of practice of chiropractic, naturopathy, and physical therapy.

XI. Massage Therapy

Background Massage is popular all over the world. The word massage has a variety of origins. It comes from the French *massage* meaning "friction of kneading", from the Arabic *massa* meaning "to touch, feel or handle," from the Latin massa meaning "mass, dough", or from the Greek verb *massō* meaning "to handle, touch, to work with the hands, to knead dough." Massage therapy appears in writings from ancient China, Japan, India, Arabic nations, Egypt, Greece, and Rome. Massage therapy (MT) was introduced in the US in the 1850s and was widely used for almost 75 years. It fell out of favor as scientific and technological advances improved medical treatment in the 1930s and 1940s (NCCAM 2013). Interest in massage was revived in the 1970s and continues to rise in popularity today. According to the 2007 National Health Interview Survey, an estimated 18 million U.S. adults and 700,000 children had received MT in the previous year (Barnes et al. 2008). In 2013, a study showed that MT was the most popular form of CAM used by children with fibromyalgia (Verkamp et al. 2013) and a separate study of two pediatric outpatient oncology clinics in Canada showed that 46.8 % of children used MT (Valji et al. 2013). A study of military children in 2011 showed that 50 % used MT (Huillet et al. 2011).

Basics Weerapong et al. noted, "Massage can provide several benefits to the body such as increased blood flow, reduced muscle tension and neurological excitability, and an increased sense of well-being" (Weerapong et al. 2005). There are many forms of massage, including deep tissue massage and Swedish massage. There are distinct forms for children known as infant and pediatric massage. According to Kulkarni et al. "Infant massage was first introduced in China in second century BC. Massaging the newborn has been a tradition in India and other Asian countries since time immemorial. Various oil-based preparations have been used depending on regional availability" (Kulkarni et al. 2010). Like infant massage, pediatric massage is also gaining popularity in the US.

Evidence Many studies have looked at MT in premature and low birth weight infants. Sunflower oil massage may be an effective and safe intervention for weight gain in low birth weight (LBW) preterm neonates (Fallah et al. 2013). MT administered to stable preterm infants was associated with higher natural killer cells and more daily weight gain (Ang et al. 2012). MT may improve growth quality of preterm male infants, and MT has the potential to improve weight gain and cause less weight loss in the first 7 days of life in LBW neonates (Kumar et al. 2013). A review article looking at massage to promote health for infants less than 6 months of age concluded that for low-risk infants, benefit was not *significant* (Bennett et al. 2013). MT may improve key pulmonary functions of children like FEV1 and FEV1/FVC ratio and lessen asthma symptoms (Fattah and Hamdy 2011). Interestingly, the anxiety level of mothers may be reduced by daily child MT, which gives mothers an active role in caring for the child (Ghazavi et al. 2010). A review article from 2011 found limited evidence for the effectiveness of massage as a symptomatic treatment of autism (Lee et al. 2011). There is some evidence to support the use of MT to improve quality of life for people living with HIV/AIDS (Hillier et al. 2010).

Safety There is limited data on the safety of MT in children. In general, MT appears to have few serious risks if performed by properly trained therapists. The number of serious injuries reported is small. Side effects of MT may include temporary discomfort, bruising, or swelling. There is also potential for sensitivity or allergic reaction to massage oils.

Education There are approximately 1,500 MT schools and training programs in the United States. An individual can investigate wether a massage training program provides a nationally recognized standard level of education by checking for accreditation by a credible agency, specifically one that follows the guidelines of the U.S. Department of Education.

Licensing of Practitioners Most states in the US require licensure for massage therapists. A few states only require certification. National certifications are administered by the National Certification Board for Therapeutic Massage and Bodywork (NCBTMB). A handful of states do not regulate massage therapists. The website for the Associated Bodywork & Massage Professionals is a resource for anyone interested in investigating regulation of massage therapists by state (MassageTherapy.com 2013).

XII. Naturopathy

Background Naturopathy originated in Germany in the early twentieth century. It is based on the belief of *vitalism*, the vital energy forces which animate bodily processes such as metabolism, reproduction, growth, and adaptation (Sarris and Wardle 2010). The term *naturopathy* is derived from Greek and Latin, and literally translates as "nature disease". Naturopathy focuses on naturally occurring substances, minimally invasive methods, and encouragement of natural healing (American Cancer Society 2008). Naturopathic practitioners in the US can be divided into three categories: traditional naturopaths, naturopathic physicians, and other health care providers that provide naturopathic services (NCCAM 2007). According to the 2007 National Health Interview Survey, which included a comprehensive survey of the use of complementary health practices by Americans, an estimated 729,000 adults and 237,000 children had used a naturopathic treatment in the previous year (Barnes et al. 2008a, b).

Basics Naturopathic practitioners treat patients based on case history, observation, medical records, and previous experience. Naturopathic treatment can include nutritional and herbal medicine, fasting, vitamins, lifestyle modification, homeopathy, Traditional Chinese Medicine, manipulation of muscles and bones, acupuncture, counseling, clinical hypnotherapy, therapeutic massage, flower essence, colonics, hydrotherapy, heat and cold applications, therapeutic exercise, and minor surgery. In general, naturopaths believe in medications and surgery but only as a last resort (Kemper 2002).

A cross-sectional survey was conducted to assess the use of naturopathic medication in children of Canada in 2008. The results showed that parents of naturopathic pediatric patients were most likely to be females, university educated, had household income >$ 60,000, and also saw a naturopathic doctor for themselves. The most common conditions for which children saw a naturopathic doctor included allergies, digestive problems, and skin problems. The most important reasons for use included using all possible options and having a more holistic approach to care. Most parents reported combining naturopathic and conventional care for their children (Leung and Verhoef 2008).

Evidence A few studies of naturopathy in children have been published. Naturopathy was shown to have benefit in cases of ear pain caused by acute otitis media (AOM) in children in which active antibiotic treatment is needed (Sarrell et al. 2003). A similar study with Otikon, an ear drop formulation of naturopathic origin, showed it to be as effective as anesthetic ear drops and was proven appropriate for the management of AOM-associated ear pain (Sarrell et al. 2001). One German study concluded that in uncomplicated AOM of childhood, an alternative treatment strategy with the natural medicine Otovowen may substantially reduce the use of antibiotics without disadvantage to the clinical outcome (Wustrow 2005). Although some of the individual therapies used in naturopathy have been studied for efficacy and safety, naturopathy as a general approach to health care has not been widely researched.

Safety Excessive fasting, dietary restrictions, or use of enemas, which are sometimes components of naturopathic treatment, may be detrimental to a person's health. Naturopathic treatment may involve taking unregulated herbs which may have harmful effects. One case report has been published about a child who sustained partial thickness burns from a garlic-petroleum jelly plaster, which had been applied at the direction of a naturopathic physician (Parish et al. 1987). Allopathic physicians should be cautioned if their patients visit naturopathic practitioners as many practitioners of naturopathy do not support routine vaccination (Halper 1981), (Lee and Kemper 2000).

Education According to the NCCAM, there are separate education paths for naturopathic physicians and traditional naturopaths. Both naturopathic physicians and traditional naturopaths sometimes refer to themselves as *naturopathic* doctors or by the abbreviation N.D. or N.M.D. Naturopathic physicians generally have completed a 4-year, graduate-level program at one of the North American naturopathic medical schools accredited by the Council on Naturopathic Medical Education, an organization recognized for accreditation purposes by the U.S. Department of Education. Traditional naturopaths, also known simply as *naturopaths*, emphasize naturopathic approaches to a healthy lifestyle, strengthening and cleansing the body, and non-invasive treatments. They do not use prescription drugs, injections, radiography, or surgery. Several schools offer training for people who want to become naturopaths, often through distance learning. Programs vary in length and content and are not accredited by organizations recognized for accreditation purposes by the U.S. Department of Education. Traditional naturopaths are not subject to licensing. Other health care providers (such as physicians, osteopathic physicians, chiropractors, dentists, and nurses) can offer naturopathic treatments and other holistic therapies, having pursued additional training in these areas, but training programs vary.

Licensure of Practitioners Seventeen states as well as the District of Columbia, Puerto Rico, and the US Virgin Islands currently license naturopathic physicians. In these jurisdictions, naturopathic physicians must graduate from a 4-year naturopathic medical college and pass an examination to receive a license. They must also fulfill annual continuing education requirements. Their scope of practice is defined by law in the state in which they practice. Some states allow naturopathic physicians to prescribe drugs, perform minor surgery, and assist in childbirth. Traditional naturopaths and other health care providers that offer naturopathic treatments are not licensed.

XIII. Osteopathy

Background Osteopathy is a philosophy and form of alternative healthcare that emphasizes the interrelationship between structure and function of the body as well as the body's ability to heal itself. Osteopaths claim to facilitate the healing process, principally by the practice of manual and manipulative therapy (AACOM 2011). Osteopathy was founded by Andrew Taylor Still in the 1860s.

Basics Osteopathic physicians follow the philosophy of holistic health. Osteopathy involves a variety of treatment modalities including osteopathic manipulative treatment (OMT), medication, surgery, exercise, and nutrition interventions. OMT is based on well recognized anatomic and physiologic principles involving the structural components of the body and their relationship. There are four major principles of osteopathy (Culbert and Olness 2009):

1. The body is a unit—an integrated unit of mind, body, and spirit
2. The body possesses self-regulatory mechanisms, having the inherent capacity to defend, repair, and remodel itself
3. Structure and function are reciprocally interrelated
4. Rational therapy is based on consideration of the first three principles

Osteopathy is commonly used in children for colic, plagiocephaly, upper respiratory infections, otitis media, asthma and a variety of neuromuscular disorders. Interest in OMT increased among general pediatricians after a session on osteopathy at the annual American Academy of Pediatrics conference in 2012 that introduced the American College of Osteopathic Pediatricians' nine-module CD-ROM entitled Pediatric Osteopathic Manipulative Treatment (POMT).

Evidence The evidence behind OMT in children is building. The results of one study of 57 children ages 6 months to 6 years of age suggest a potential benefit of OMT as adjuvant therapy in children with recurrent acute otitis media (AOM). OMT may prevent or decrease surgical intervention or antibiotic overuse (Mills et al. 2003). A different study that looked at Echinacea purpurea supplementation and/or OMT for prevention of otitis media (OM) showed that there may be increased risk of OM with Echinacea purpurea and no difference in risk with a regimen of up to five OMT's in prevention of OM (Wahl et al. 2008). A pilot study with children with cerebral palsy and chronic constipation suggests that osteopathic methods may be helpful as an alternative treatment for constipation (Tarsuslu et al. 2009). Another study showed that a series of treatments using osteopathy in the cranial field and/or myofascial release improved motor function in children with moderate to severe spastic cerebral palsy (Duncan et al. 2008). A related study showed that neurologic performance significantly improved after 6–12 OMTs in children with diagnosed neurologic problems and to a lesser degree in children with medical or structural diagnoses. One study in the UK of children with cerebral palsy found no statistically significant evidence that cranial osteopathy leads to sustained improvement in motor function, pain, sleep or quality of life in children aged 5–12 years with cerebral palsy (Wyatt et al. 2011). A randomized controlled trial in children looked at the therapeutic relevance of OMT in the pediatric asthma population. The OMT group showed a statistically significant improvement in peak expiratory flow rates suggesting that OMT has a therapeutic effect among this patient population (Guiney et al. 2005).

Although individual studies have shown benefit of OMT in pediatric conditions, a systematic review was published in the Journal of Pediatrics in 2013 by Posadzki et al. which showed that "the evidence of the effectiveness of OMT for pediatric conditions remains unproven due to the paucity and low methodological quality of the primary studies "(Posadzki et al. 2013)". The Osteopathic Research Center in Texas is the premier research center focusing on the clinical efficacy and mechanisms of action of OMT (Osteopathic Research Center 2012).

Safety Osteopathy is safe for babies, children and adolescents if practiced by an experienced, licensed practitioner.

Education There are currently 30 colleges of osteopathic medicine, offering instruction at 40 locations in 28 states (AACOM 2011). Osteopathic physicians attend a 4-year program and earn the degree of Doctor of Osteopathic Medicine (D.O.), a degree equivalent to that of Doctor of Medicine (M.D.) (AMA 2013).

Licensing of Practitioners Doctors of Osteopathy are licensed by each individual state as are Doctors of Medicine.

XIV. Reiki

Background Reiki, Japanese for "spiritually guided life force energy," is believed to have originated nearly 2500 years ago in Tibet. This ancient therapy had been forgotten until Dr Mikao Usui renewed its implementation in 1922. Reiki treats the whole person including body, emotions, mind, and spirit. It creates beneficial effects including relaxation and feelings of peace, security, and wellbeing. It is believed that if a person's "life force energy" is low, then that person is more likely to become ill, and if it is high, the person is more likely to be healthy (Reiki 2013). In 2007, the NCCAM survey revealed that 0.5 % of United States adults used Reiki therapy (NCCAM 2013). According to the American Hospital Association, approximately 15 % (800 hospitals) in the United States offer Reiki therapy to their patients (Gill 2008).

Basics Reiki practice involves gentle laying of hands (or by distant practice) by a trained Reiki practitioner. Reiki practitioners place themselves in a meditative state whereby energy flows through the palms from practitioner to patient. It is implied that this transfer of energy restores equilibrium and heals the patient (vanderVaart et al. 2009).

Evidence Much of the Reiki therapeutic research literature has relied on relatively small case studies. Preliminary research suggests Reiki to be helpful in stress reduction; decreasing anxiety; promoting well being; decreasing perioperative anxiety, pain, and cancer-related pain; and decreasing fatigue. There has been limited documentation of Reiki's effect on biological stress markers such as blood pressure, salivary cortisol, and immune globulin A. However, subjective psychological measures imply that Reiki decreases anxiety. It is a therapy which can be self taught, is inexpensive, and may be beneficial for the psychosocial well-being of patients and families within a stressful hospital setting. A review study in 2013 concluded that therapeutic implementation of Reiki could not be substantiated given the poor quality of existing studies. The authors stated that this conclusion does not imply that Reiki is not beneficial for individual patients, as individual benefit has been noted in anecdotal studies. The authors also noted that studies using Reiki Master practitioners had an overall significant improvement in measured outcomes (Kundu et al. 2013). Randomized controlled studies are emerging within Reiki models. Researchers at Yale recently conducted a randomized trial involving a 49 heart attack patients to ascertain if Reiki treatment would affect heart rate variability (HRV). Patients were randomized to receive a 20-min Reiki session, classical music, or resting control. A Likert 10-point scale was used to query emotional states. The mean HRV increased statistically from baseline in the Reiki group ($p=0.02$), which was greater than the music group ($p=0.007$). Reiki therapy was also noted to have an increase in positive emotions on the Likert scale (Friedman et al. 2010).

Kundu et al. investigated whether a Reiki training program for families was feasible at Seattle Children's Hospital. Seventeen families agreed to the study, and sessions were taught by a Reiki Master. Sixty-five percent of families attended 3 Reiki training sessions. Seventy-six percent of families stated that Reiki training provided increased comfort for their child, 88% described improved relaxation, and 41% claimed pain relief benefit. All participants noted that the Reiki training provided them with a way to actively participate in their child's hospital care, and overall, the program was well received (Kundu et al. 2013).

Safety Reiki appears to be generally safe, and no serious side effects have been reported (NCCAM 2013).

Education Reiki typically involves three levels of training. Level I Reiki focuses on the practitioner learning hands-on treatment of self and others. Level II encourages a deeper understanding of healing energy flow, and the practitioner learns to incorporate distant healing. Level III, or Reiki Master, focuses on further inner spiritual development and may teach the practice of Reiki. All levels of training involve "attunement" by a Reiki Master, which involves a flow of energy from the Reiki practitioner to the patient.

Licensing of Practitioners There are no state licensure requirements for Reiki practitioners. Reiki practitioners are trained by a Reiki Master and are apprenticed. There are no national certifying examinations (Kemper et al. 2012).

XV. Therapeutic Touch

Background Therapeutic touch (TT) was developed by Dr Dolores Krieger, nursing professor at New York University, and Dora Kunz, a theosophy professor, for use in the nursing field as a method of energy exchange to facilitate healing. The Therapeutic Touch International Association defines TT as "a holistic, evidence-based therapy that incorporates the intentional and compassionate use of universal energy to promote balance and well-being" (TTIA 2014).

Basics Typical TT sessions have four phases and last a total of 20 min. The patient is fully clothed in a sitting or lying position. In the first phase, practitioners center their own mind, body, and emotion for centering of self. In the second phase, practitioners place their hands 2–6 inches away from the patient in order to sense the patient's energy field. This is a dynamic process where practitioners move their hands in a rhythmic manner from the patient's head to their feet. The third phase involves clearing and rebalancing the recipient's energy field. The fourth phase involves evaluation and session cessation (Culbert and Olness 2009).

Evidence Most adult and pediatric studies have been anecdotal, small case studies, with randomization, statistical, and methodological limitations. Overall, there may be support for reduction of anxiety following TT sessions. One small pilot study in preterm infants showed that heart period variability was increased positively for the

TT group compared with the non-TT group. The study revealed no adverse effects of TT in preterm infants (Whitley and Rich 2008). Kemper and Kelly found that pediatric patients received TT for a variety of reasons including anxiety, fatigue, insomnia, and pain. Some pain conditions included abdominal pain, headache, postoperative pain, cancer pain, and fibromyalgia. The authors noted that these patients consistently responded to TT sessions and that there were no adverse events (Kemper and Kelly 2004). Interestingly, TT may have an effect *in vitro*. Gronowicz et al. studied the effects of TT on the proliferation of normal human cells. They observed a significant increase in the proliferation of fibroblasts, osteoblasts, and tenocytes in culture. TT appears to increase human osteoblast DNA synthesis, differentiation, and mineralization, and to decrease differentiation and mineralization in a human osteosarcoma-derived cell line. (Gronowicz et al. 2008).

Safety According to the American Cancer Society, TT is generally considered safe when performed by trained professionals. Some of the reported side effects include nausea, dizziness, restlessness, and irritability. Relying on TT alone and delaying or avoiding conventional medical care for serious medical problems may have serious health consequences (ACS 2013).

Education TT is taught in more than 70 US nursing and medical schools and in almost 100 countries worldwide.

Licensing of Practitioners TT practitioners do not need formal licensing. There is no national certifying examination.

XVI. Traditional Chinese Medicine

Background Traditional Chinese medicine (TCM) is rooted in the ancient philosophy of Taoism and dates back more than 5000 years. TCM encompasses many different practices like use of herbs and acupuncture and is practiced side by side with Western medicine in many of China's hospitals and clinics.

Basics According to the *Huang Di Nei Jing* (Inner Canon of the Yellow Emperor), the classic Chinese medicine text, there are eight chief principles to analyze symptoms and categorize conditions: cold/heat, interior/exterior, excess/deficiency, and yin/yang. TCM also uses the theory of five elements—fire, earth, metal, water, and wood—to explain how the body works; these elements correspond to particular organs and tissues in the body. TCM emphasizes individualized treatment. Practitioners traditionally used four methods to evaluate a patient's condition: observing (especially the tongue), hearing/smelling, asking/interviewing, and touching/palpating (especially the pulse). TCM practitioners use a variety of therapies in an effort to promote health and treat disease. The most commonly used are Chinese herbal medicine and acupuncture (NCCAM 2013; ACTCM 2013).

Evidence Despite the widespread use of TCM in China and in the West, scientific evidence of its effectiveness is limited. TCM's complexity and underlying conceptual foundations present challenges for researchers seeking evidence on whether and how it works. Most research has focused on specific modalities, primarily acupuncture and common Chinese herbal remedies. A 2013 review of the literature about safety and efficiency of acupuncture therapy in term and preterm infants included 6 studies. The data suggested that acupuncture could be a safe nonpharmacologic treatment option for pain reduction in term and preterm infants and could also be a nonpharmacologic treatment option for infantile colic (Raith et al. 2013). A group in New York reviewed the literature for TCM in allergic diseases in children and concluded that TCM therapy including herbal medicines and acupuncture for allergic disorders in children is well tolerated (Li 2009). One study group is investigating an herbal formula with a high safety profile known as FAHF-2. FAHF-2 has been shown to prevent anaphylaxis in murine models of food allergy. Early clinical trials demonstrate the safety and tolerability of this formula in individuals with food allergies. An ongoing Phase II clinical trial will evaluate the efficacy of FAHF-2 in protecting individuals from allergen-induced allergic reactions during oral food challenges (Yang and Chiang 2013; Wang 2013). In China, a nationwide population-based study analyzed a cohort of 1 million randomly sampled patients in Taiwan to look at children with asthma using TCM. The most commonly prescribed TCM formula was Ding-chuan-tang, or Xing-ren (Semen Armeniacae Amarum) for the single herb (Huang et al. 2013). A similar study in China from a nationwide database review of children and asthma showed that the Ma-Xing-Gan-Shi-Tang (MXGST) was the most commonly used herbal formula, followed by Xiao-Qing-Long-Tang (13.1%) and Xing-Su-San (12.8%). Zhe Bei Mu is the most frequently used single herb (14.6%), followed by Xing Ren (10.7%) (Chen et al. 2013). Ningdong granule is commonly used in China to treat ADHD. Li et al. looked at ADHD in 2011 and noted that "Compared to methylphenidate, Ningdong granule is effective and safe for ADHD children in the short term…and promises to be an alternative medication, safely and effectively" (Li et al. 2011). A Cochrane database review showed that current evidence does not support the use of acupuncture for treatment of autism spectrum disorders (ASD). There is no conclusive evidence that acupuncture is effective for treatment of ASD in children, and no RCTs have been carried out with adults (Cheuk et al. 2011). A Cochrane review of studies by Cheuk et al. of insomnia and acupuncture with patients ages 15–98 showed that "due to poor methodological quality, high levels of heterogeneity and publication bias, the current evidence is not sufficiently rigorous to support or refute acupuncture for treating insomnia. Larger high-quality clinical trials are required" (Cheuk et al. 2011). A study from Egypt showed that acupuncture treatment in patients with primary nocturnal enuresis appears effective in increasing the percentage of dry nights, with stable results even after the end of treatment courses (El Koumi et al. 2013).

Acupuncture research has produced a large body of scientific evidence. Studies suggest that it may be useful for a number of different conditions, but additional research is needed.

Although there is evidence that herbs may be effective for some conditions, most studies have been methodologically flawed, and additional, better designed research is needed before any conclusions can be drawn (NCCAM 2013).

Safety TCM herbal medicines are generally marketed in the United States as dietary supplements. Not all Chinese herbal products are safe for all. There have been reports of products being contaminated with toxins or heavy metals and many do not contain the listed ingredients. Some of the herbs used in Chinese medicine can interact with allopathic drugs, can have serious side effects, or may be unsafe for people with certain medical conditions (NCCAM 2013). A systematic review of 37 studies concluded that needle acupuncture is safe for children when it is performed by appropriately trained practitioners who follow detailed protocols (Adams et al. 2011). Currently, acupuncture in infants should be limited to clinical trials and studies evaluating short- and long-term effects and should be performed only by practitioners with adequate training and experience in neonatal/pediatric acupuncture (Raith et al. 2013).

Education There are more than 50 master's programs for acupuncture and Oriental medicine in the United States. Most states allow conventional medical doctors and chiropractors to practice acupuncture with little or no formal training.

Licensing of Practitioners The National Certification Commission for Acupuncture and Oriental Medicine (NCCAOM) offers national board certification in TCM. Practitioners must complete at least 3 years of full-time education before becoming eligible for national certification. All but a few states have regulations in place concerning the practice of acupuncture. This usually includes licensing requirements for non-MD practitioners and specifications on scope of practice for MDs and other health professionals. Most states require national board certification as a prerequisite for state certification or licensure. State requirements vary but contact information for each state can be found at acupuncture.com.

The American College of Traditional Chinese Medicine has a directory of practitioners which lists pediatric specialists.

XVII. Yoga

Background Yoga is a mind-body practice that originated in the Hindu tradition in India around 5000 BCE (Samuel 2008). The word "yoga" comes from Sanskrit meaning "to yoke" or to unite the body, mind, and spirit. Yoga has evolved over time but continues to focus on these important connections. On a philosophical level, yoga is a manner of achieving *oneness* with oneself, with a higher being, or with God. In 2007, there were over 1.5 million pediatric yoga users in the U.S.(Nahin et al. 2009; Barnes et al. 2007). Within popular culture, yoga is perceived as a way to develop and maintain a healthy mind and body. For adults, yoga is commonly taught in gyms, spas, yoga studios, and colleges. There is increasing interest in yoga for babies, children, and adolescents. Yoga classes are now offered for children in yoga studios, some especially designed for children. Research has shown that school curriculums incorporating stress management programs improve academic performance, self-esteem, classroom behaviors, concentration, and emotional balance. In addition, there is a decrease in helplessness, aggression, and behavioral problems of students (Kiselika et al. 1994; Manjunath and Telles 2004). Many school districts have considered incorporating yoga into their P.E. programs. The Encinitas, California school district gained a San Diego Superior Court judge's approval to use yoga in P.E., holding against the parents who claimed the practice was intrinsically religious and hence should not be part of a state-funded program (NY Times 2013). School teachers are opting to introduce yoga into their daily school routine. One curriculum available to teachers is known as YogaKids Tools for Schools-Breathe Life into Learning. This curriculum uses a DVD, flashcards with yoga poses, and relaxation stories to calm children (Yogakids 2013).

Basics Yoga consists of breathing (pranayama), postures (asanas), and meditation or relaxation. Yoga can be an effective training for children and adolescents, including those with special needs. It is a form of physical exercise that can help with breathing, flexibility, focus, mindfulness, and stress relief. Children are often intrigued by the idea that many yoga poses are based on animals and the different postures that the animals perform in nature.

Evidence Individual studies have shown benefit of yoga in children. Yoga has been used to improve posture among children with physical malformations (Savic et al. 1990) and to treat anxiety in child and adolescent psychiatric patients (Platania-Solazzo 1992). Yoga has been found to improve children's hyperactive and inattentive behaviour, self-esteem and relationship quality with parents (Peck et al. 2005). One study showed that yoga can be beneficial for patients with attention-deficit/hyperactivity disorder (ADHD) even when performed from a videotaped lesson (Harrison et al. 2004). Yoga has been found to decrease physiological anxiety among children with vision impairments (Telles and Srinivas 1998). Yoga exercises in adolescents with childhood asthma can result in an increase in pulmonary function and exercise capacity (Jain et al. 1991). A published abstract reported positive illness perception results of a 4-month yoga protocol among a small group of young adults (aged 15–22 years) with irritable bowel syndrome (IBS) (Raghavan et al. 2000). Kuttner showed that yoga has proven useful in adolescents with IBS (Kuttner et al. 2006). One study showed an overall reduction in both pain and anxiety scores with yoga in a small sample of pediatric hematology-oncology patients. The focus was on sickle cell patients in vaso-occlusive crisis as well as inpatient and outpatient pediatric oncology patients (Moody et al. 2009). A systematic review conducted in 2009 concluded that there is limited data on the clinical applications of yoga among the pediatric population. Most published controlled trials were suggestive of benefit, but results are preliminary based on low quantity and quality of trials. Preliminary evidence showed that yoga might be beneficial for children's physical fitness, but the researchers believed that studies should be conducted in different cultural settings to evaluate the feasibility of yoga as a form of exercise for children. Studies are also needed to examine applications of yoga to improve pediatric behavior and development, such as in the case of kids with ADHD or other mental health conditions. Further research of yoga for children by using a higher standard of methodology and reporting is warranted (Birdee et al. 2009).

Safety Yoga is generally considered to be safe for children. It is a low-impact activity. Like any exercise, gentle stretching is recommended before the activity. Of note, the American Yoga Association does not recommend yoga for children younger than 16 years of age because their bodies' nervous and glandular systems are still growing, and the effect of yoga exercises on these systems may interfere with natural growth. There are no available studies documenting the validity of this concern.

Education There are hundreds of yoga schools and institutes across the world. The education is not standardized. The Yoga Alliance is the largest nonprofit association representing yoga teachers, schools and studios in the U.S. The Yoga Alliance Registry is a registry of teachers and schools whose training meets the standards of the Yoga Alliance. Teachers who have completed specialized training to teach yoga to children are eligible to become a Registered Children's Yoga Teacher through the Yoga Alliance (Yoga Alliance 2013).

Licensing of Practitioners The US government does not promote a licensing policy for yoga practitioners. To join the professional provider network of the Integrative Medicine and Holistic Health Association, yoga teachers must complete 500 h of training and yoga therapists must complete 700 h of training. Practitioners and schools can voluntarily join the Yoga Alliance which promotes standards of education and practice. A special license for practitioners who teach yoga to special-needs children is the Yoga for the Special Child®, LLC license (Yoga for the Special Child 2013).

References

Aase K, Blaakær J (2013) [Chiropractic care of infants with colic lacks evidence], [Article in Danish]. Ugeskr Laeger 175(7):424–428

ACA-American Chiropractic Association (2009) Policy statement on vaccination. http://www.acatoday.org/level2_css.cfm?t1id=10&t2id=117. Accessed 11 Dec 2013

ACAOM- Accreditation Commission for Acupuncture and Oriental Medicine (2014) http://www.acaom.org. Accessed 17 Jan 2014

ACS- American Cancer Society (2013) http://www.cancer.org/treatment/treatmentsandsideeffects/complementaryandalternativemedicine/mindbodyandspirit/biofeedback. Accessed 1 May 2014

Acupuncture.com (2013) http://www.acupuncture.com/statelaws/statelaw.htm. Accessed 1 Dec 2013

Adams D, Cheng F, Jou H et al (2011) The safety of pediatric acupuncture: a systematic review. Pediatrics 128(6):e1575–1587. doi:10.1542/peds.2011-1091. Epub 2011 Nov 21

Adams D, Dagenais S, Clifford T et al (2013) Complementary and alternative medicine use by pediatric specialty outpatients. Pediatrics 131(2):225–232

Aggarwal B, Harikumar K (2009) Potential therapeutic effects of curcumin, the anti-inflammatory agent, against neurodegenerative, cardiovascular, pulmonary, metabolic, autoimmune and neoplastic diseases. Int J Biochem Cell Biol 41(1):40–59

AIA- Alliance of International (2013) Aromatherapists http://www.alliance-aromatherapists.org/education/aromatherapy-schools/. Accessed 17 Dec 2013

Alcantara J, Adamek R (2012) The chiropractic care of a child with extremity tremors concomitant with a medical diagnosis of conversion disorder. Complement Ther Clin Pract 18(2):89–93

Alcantara J, Alcantara JD, Alcantara J (2011) A systematic review of the literature on the chiropractic care of patients with autism spectrum disorder. Explore (NY) 7(6):384–390

Alfaleh K, Anabrees J, Bassler D et al (2011) Probiotics for prevention of necrotizing enterocolitis in preterm infants. Cochrane Database Syst Rev 16(3):CD005496

Allen S, Martinez E, Gregorio G et al (2010) Probiotics for treating acute infectious diarrhoea. Cochrane Database of Syst Rev 10(11):CD003048

Altunc U, Pittler MH, Ernst E (2007) Homeopathy for childhood and adolescence ailments: systematic review of randomized clinical trials. Mayo Clinic Proc 81(1):69–75

AMA (American Medical Association) (2011) Medicine, American Medical Association. http://www.ama-assn.org/ama1/pub/upload/mm/40/physician.pdf. Accessed 11 Feb 2013

Ambartsumyan L, Nurko S (2013) Review of organic causes of fecal incontinence in children: evaluation and treatment. Expert Rev Gastroenterol Hepatol 7(7):657–667. doi:10.1586/1747 4124.2013.832500

American Cancer Society (2008) Naturopathic medicine. http://www.cancer.org/treatment/treatmentsandsideeffects/complementaryandalternativemedicine/mindbodyandspirit/naturopathicmedicine. Accessed 26 Nov 2013

American College of Traditional Chinese Medicine (2013) http://www.actcm.edu/. Accessed 12 Jan 2013

American Society of Clinical Hypnosis (ASCH) (2014) https://www.asch.net/Public/GeneralInfoonHypnosis/DefinitionofHypnosis.aspx. Accessed 10 Jan 2014

Amsterdam JD, Li Y, Soeller I, Rockwell K et al (2009) A randomized, double-blind, placebo controlled trial of oral Matricaria recutita (chamomille) extract therapy of generalized anxiety disorder. J Clin Psychopharmacol 29(4):378–382

Anbar R (2012) Functional respiratory disorders. Springer, New York

Ang JY, Lua JL, Mathur A et al (2012) A randomized placebo-controlled trial of massage therapy on the immune system of preterm infants. Pediatrics 130(6):e1549–1558

Arns M, Derldder S, Strehl U et al (2009) Efficacy of neurofeedback treatment in ADHD: the effects of inattention, impulsivity, and hyperactivity: a meta-analysis. Clin EEG Neurosci 40(3):180–189

Athavale VB (2013) Bala Veda. Chaukhamba Sanskrit Pratishthan Oriental Publishers. New Delhi

Badar VA, Thawani VR, Wakode PT et al (2005) Efficacy of Tinospora cordifolia in allergic rhinitis. J Ethnopharmacol 96(3):445–449

Bailey RL, Gahche JJ, Miller PE et al (2013) Why US adults use dietary supplements. JAMA Intern Med 173(5):355–361

Barnes PM, Bloom B, Nahin RL, (2007) Complementary and alternative medicine use among adults and children: United States

Barnes PM, Bloom B, Nahin R (2008b) CDC national health statistics report #12. Complementary and alternative medicine use among adults and children: United States.12:1–23

Barnes PM, Bloom B, Nahin RL (2008a) Complementary and alternative medicine use among adults and children: United States, 2007. Natl Health Stat Report (12):1–23

Barrett B, Brown R, Rakel D et al (2011) Placebo effects and the common cold: a randomized controlled trial. Ann Fam Med 9(4):312–322

BCIA -Biofeedback Certification International Alliance (2013) http://www.bcia.org/i4a/pages/index.cfm?pageid=3350. Accessed 1 May 2014

Becker B, Kuhn U, Hardewig-Budny B (2006) Double-blind, randomized evaluation of clinical efficacy and tolerability of an apple pectin-chamomille extract in children with unspecific diarrhea. Arzneimittelforschung 56:387–393

Bennett C, Underdown A, Barlow J (2013) Massage for promoting mental and physical health in typically developing infants under the age of six months. Cochrane Database Syst Rev 4:CD005038

Birdee GS, Yeh GY, Wayne PM, Phillips RS, Davis RB, Gardiner P (2009) Clinical applications of yoga for the pediatric population: a systematic review. Acad Pediatr 9(4):212–220.e1–9

Bothe DA, Grignon JB, Olness KN (2014) The effects of a stress management intervention in elementary school children. J Dev Behav Pediatr 35(1):62–67. doi:10.1097/DBP.0000000000000016

Budzynska K, Gardner ZE, Dugoua J-J et al (2012) Systematic review of breastfeeding and medicine. Breastfeed Med 7(6):489–503

Buscemi N, Vandermeer B, Hooton N et al (2005) The efficacy and safety of exogenous melatonin for primary sleep disorders: a meta-analysis. J Gen Intern Med 20(12):1151–1158

Canani RB, Cirillo P, Terrin G et al (2007) Probiotics for treatment of acute diarrhoea in children: randomized clinical trial of five different preparations. BMJ 335(7615):340

Capello G, Spezzaferro M, Grossi L et al (2007) Peppermint oil (Mintoil) in the treatment of irritable bowel syndrome: a prospective double blind placebo-controlled randomized trial. Dig Liver Dis 39(6):530–536

Carson CF, Hammer KAR (2006) Melaleuca alternifolia (Tea Tree) oil: a review of antimicrobial and other medicinal properties. Clin Microbiol Rev 19(1):50–62

Charrois T, Hrudey J Gardiner P et al (2006) Peppermint oil. Pediatr Rev 27:e49–e51

Charrois T, Sadler C, Vohra S (2007) Complementary, holistic, and integrative medicine: St. John's wort. Pediatr Rev 28:69–72

Chen HY, Lin YH, Thien PF et al (2013) Identifying core herbal treatments for children with asthma: implication from a Chinese herbal medicine database in taiwan. Evid Based Complement Alternat Med 2013(2013):125943.

Cheuk DK, Wong V, Chen WX (2011) Acupuncture for autism spectrum disorders (ASD). Cochrane Database Syst Rev (9):CD007849.

Cheuk DK, Yeung WF, Chung KF et al (2012) Acupuncture for insomnia. Cochrane Database Syst Rev 9:CD005472

Chiou E, Nurko S (2010) Management of functional abdominal pain and irritable bowel syndrome in children and adolescents. Expert Rev Gastroenterol Hepatol 4(3):293–304

Cohen HA, Varsano I, Kahan E et al (2004) Effectiveness of an herbal preparation containing Echinacea, Propolis, and vitamin C in preventing respiratory tract infections in children: a randomized, double-blind, placebo controlled multicenter study. Arch Pediatr Adolesc Med 158:217–221

ConsumerLab (2013) www.consumerlabs.com. Accessed 1 March 2014

ConsumerLab.com. Product Review (2002) Echinacea. umm.edu/health/medical/altmed/herb/echinacea. Accessed 1 Feb 2014

Council on Chiropractic Education (2007) Standards for doctor of chiropractic programs and requirements for institutional status. http://www.cce-usa.org/uploads/2007_January_STANDARDS.pdf. Accessed 17 Dec 2013

Culbert T, Olness K (2009) Integrative pediatrics. Oxford University Press, New York, pp 192–203, 341 (Well Intergrative Medicine Library)

Danno K, Colas A, Masson JL et al (2013). Homeopathic treatment of migraine in children: results of a prospective, multicenter, observational study. J Altern Complement Med 19(2):119–123

DerMarderosian A (ed) (1996) Melatonin. In: The Review of Natural Products. St. Louis, Mo: Facts and Comparisons, Inc

Deshpande G, Rao S, Patole S et al (2010) Updated meta-analysis of probiotics for preventing necrotizing enterocolitis in preterm neonates. Pediatrics 125(5):921–930

Dobson D, Lucassen PL, Miller JJ et al (2012) Manipulative therapies for infantile colic. Cochrane Database Syst Rev 12:CD004796

Duncan B, McDonough-Means S, Worden K et al (2008) Effectiveness of osteopathy in the cranial field and myofascial release versus acupuncture as complementary treatment for children with spastic cerebral palsy: a pilot study. J Am Osteopath Assoc 108(10):559–570

Durand VM, Barlow D (2009) Abnormal psychology: an iintegrative approach. Wadsworth Cengage Learning, Belmont, p 331

Edris AE (2007) Pharmaceutical and therapeutic Potentials of essential oils and their individual volatile constituents: a review. Phytother Res 21(4):308–323

El Koumi MA, Ahmed SA, Salama AM (2013) Acupuncture efficacy in the treatment of persistent primary nocturnal enuresis. Arab J Nephrol Transplant 6(3):173–176

Elder JS, Diaz M (2013) Vesicoureteral reflux-the role of bladder and bowel dysfunction. Nat Rev Urol 10(11):640–648. doi:10.1038/nrurol.221. Epub 2013 Oct 15

Elseify MY, Mohammed NH, Alsharkawy AA, Elseoudy ME (2013) Laser acupuncture in treatment of childhood bronchial asthma. J Complement Integr Med 10. pii://j/jcim.2013.10.issue-1/jcim-2012-0006/jcim-2012-0006.xml. doi:10.1515/jcim-2012-0006

Ernst E (2005) Is homeopathy a clinically valuable approach? Trends Pharmacol Sci 26(11):547–548

Fallah R, Akhavan Karbasi S, Golestan M et al (2013) Sunflower oil versus no oil moderate pressure massage leads to greater increases in weight in preterm neonates who are low birth weight. Early Hum Dev 89(9):769–772

Ferrance RJ, Miller J (2010) Chiropractic diagnosis and management of non-musculoskeletal conditions in children and adolescents. Chiropr Osteopat 18:14

Fitzgerald M, Culbert T, Finkelstein M et al (2007) The effect of gender and ethnicity on children's attitudes and preferences for essential oils: a pilot study. Explore (NY) 3(4):378–385

Forbes RJ (1970) A short history of the art of distillation. E.J. Brill, Leiden

Ford A, Talley N (2008) The effect of fibre, antispasmotics, and peppermint oil in the treatment of irritable bowel syndrome: a systematic review and meta analysis. BMJ 337:a2313

Fowler NA (2006) Aromatherapy, used as an integrative tool for crisis management by adolescents in a residential treatment center. J Child Adolesc Psychiatr Nurs 19(2):69–76

Frei H, Thurneysen A (2001a) Homeopathy in acute otitis media in children: treatment effect or spontaneous resolution? Br Homeopath J 90(4):180–182

Frei H, Thurneysen A (2001b) Treatment for hyperactive children: homeopathy and methylphenidate compared in a family setting. Br Homeopath J 90(4):183–188

Friedman R, Burg M, Miles P et al (2010) Effects of Reiki on autonomic activity early after acute coronary syndrome. J Am Coll Cardiol 56(12):995–996

Frymann VM, Carney RE, Springall P (1992) Effect of osteopathic medical management on neurologic development in children. J Am Osteopath Assoc 92(6):729–744

Gardiner P (2007) Complementary, holistic and integrative medicine: Chamomille. Pediatr Rev 28:e16–e18

Gardiner P, Graham R, Legedza AT et al (2007) Factors associated with herbal therapy use by adults in the United States. Altern Ther Health Med 13(2):22–29

Gevensleben H et al (2009) Is neurofeedback an efficacious treatment for ADHD? A randomized controlled clinical trial. J Child Psychol Psychiatry 50(7):780–789

Ghazavi Z, Namnabati M, Faghihinia J et al (2010) Effects of massage therapy of asthmatic children on the anxiety level of mothers. Iran J Nurs Midwifery Res Summer 15(3):130–134

Gill L (2008) More hospitals offer alternative therapies for mind, body, spirit. USA Today. http://www.reiki.org/reikinews/reiki_in_hospitals.html. Accessed 5 Jan 2014

Glossary of Osteopathic Terminology (2011) Educational Council on Osteopathic Principles (ECOP). American Association of Colleges of Osteopathic Medicine (AACOM). http://www.aacom.org/resources/bookstore/Pages/glossary.aspx. Accessed 24 Nov 2013

Goodyer J, Gunther RT (eds) (1959) The greek herbal of dioscorides. Hafner Publishing, New York

Gronowicz GA, Jhaveri A, Clarke LW et al (2008) Therapeutic touch stimulates the proliferation of human cells in culture. J Altern Complement Med 14(3):233–239

Guiney PA, Chou R, Vianna A et al (2005) Effects of osteopathic manipulative treatment on pediatric patients with asthma: a randomized controlled trial. J Am Osteopath Assoc 105(1):7–12

Hahnemann S (1833) The homœopathic medical doctrine, or "Organon of the Healing Art". Dublin: W. F. Wakeman. pp iii, 48–49

Halper J, Berger LR (1981) Naturopaths and childhood immunizations: heterodoxy among the unorthodox. Pediatrics 68(3):407–410

Hanai H, Iida T, Takeuchi K (2006) Curcumin maintenance therapy for ulcerative colitis: randomized, multicenter, double-blind, placebo controlled trial. Clin Gastroenterol Hepatol 4(12):1502–1506

Harrison LJ, Manocha R, Rubia KS (2004) yoga meditation as a family treatment programme for children with Attention Deficit-Hyperactivity Disorder. Clin Child Psychol Psychiatry 9:479–497

Healing Touch Program (2013) http://www.healingtouchprogram.com/about/founder-s-story. Accessed 4 Jan 2014

Health Canada (2003) Natural health products regulations SOR/2003-196. http://gazette.gc.ca/archives/p2/2003/2003-06-18/html/sor-dors196-eng.html. [Feb 17; 2012], Canada Gazette. 2003 137(13)

Hempel S, Newberry S, Maher A et al (2012) Probiotics for the prevention and treatment of antibiotic-associated diarrhea: a systematic review and meta-analysis. JAMA 307(18):1959–1969

Hestbaek L, Stochkendahl MJ (2010) The evidence base for chiropractic treatment of musculoskeletal conditions in children and adolescents: The emperor's new suit? Chiropr Osteopat 18:15. doi:10.1186/1746-1340-18-15

Hillier SL, Louw Q, Morris L et al (2010) Massage therapy for people with HIV/AIDS. Cochrane Database Syst Rev (1):CD007502

Hoebert M, van der Heijden KB, van Geijlswijk IM et al (2009) Long-term follow up of melatonin treatment in children with ADHD and chronic sleep onset insomnia. J Pineal Res 47:1–7

Huang T, Shu X, Huang YS et al (2011) Complementary and miscellaneous interventions for nocturnal enuresis in children. Cochrane Database Syst Rev 184(8):908–911

Huang TP, Liu PH, Lien AS et al (2013) Characteristics of traditional Chinese medicine use in children with asthma: a nationwide population-based study. Allergy 68(12):1610–1613

Hubbard TA, Crisp CA (2010) Cessation of cyclic vomiting in a 7-year-old girl after upper cervical chiropractic care: a case report. J Chiropr Med 9(4):179–183

Huillet A, Erdie-Lalena C, Norvell D et al (2011) Complementary and alternative medicine used by children in military pediatric clinics. J Altern Complement Med 17(6):531–537

Humphreys BK (2010) Possible adverse events in children treated by manual therapy: a review. Chiropr Osteopat 18:12

Hyams JS, Burke G, Davis PM et al (1996) Abdominal pain and irritable bowel syndrome in adolescents: a community-based study. J Pediatr 129(2):220–226

ICA Policy Statements (2013) http://www.chiropractic.org/?p=ica/policies. Accessed 17 Dec 2013

Jafarzadeh M, Arman S, Pour FF (2013) Effect of aromatherapy with orange essential oil on salivary cortisol and pulse rate in children during dental treatment: a randomized controlled clinical trial. Adv Biomed Res 2:10

Jain SC, Rai L, Valecha A, Jha UK, Bhatnager SOD, Ram K (1991) Effect of yoga training on exercise tolerance in adolescents with childhood asthma. J Asthma 28:437–442

Jean D, Cyr C (2007) Use of complementary and alternative medicine in a general pediatric clinic. Pediatrics 120:e138–141

Josey ES, Tackett RL (1999) St. John's wort: a new alternative for depression? Int J Clin Pharmacol Ther 37(3):111–119

Joswick D (2014) Acufinder- How does acupuncture work? https://www.acufinder.com/Acupuncture+Information/Detail/How+does+acupuncture+work+. Accessed 17 Jan 2014

Karande S, Sholapurwala R (2013) Ayurveda for the management of dyslexia in children: Some caution required. Ayu 34(1):131. doi:10.4103/0974-8520.115434

Karlson G, Bennicke P (2013) Acupuncture in asthmatic children: a prospective, randomized, controlled clinical trial of efficacy. Altern Ther Health Med 19(4):13–19

Karpouzis F, Bonello R, Pollard H (2010) Chiropractic care for paediatric and adolescent Attention-Deficit/Hyperactivity Disorder: a systematic review. Chiropr Osteopat 18:13

Kasper S, Anghelescu IG, Szegedi A et al (2006) Superior efficacy of St. John's wort extract WS 5570 compared to placebo in patients with major depression: a randomized, double-blind, placebo controlled, multi-center trial. BMC Med 2006(4):14

Kasper S, Caraci F, Forti B et al (2010) Efficacy and tolerability of Hypericum extract for the treatment of mild to moderate depression. Eur Neuropsychopharmacol 20(11):747–765

Kemper KJ (1996) Seven herbs every pediatrician should know. Contemp Pediatr 13(12):79–91

Kemper KJ (2002) The holistic pediatrician, harper collins, 2nd edn. HarperQuill, ISBN-13: 978-0060084271 p 16–17

Kemper KJ (2010) Mental health, naturally. American Academy of Pediatrics. Elk Grove Village, IL. ISBN 978-1-58110-310-6

Kemper K, Kelly K (2004) Treating children with TT and Healing Touch. Pediatr Ann 33(4):249–252

Kemper KJ, Vohra S, Walls R (2008) Task force on complementary and alternative medicine; provisional section on complementary, holistic, and integrative medicine. American Academy of Pediatrics. The use of complementary and alternative medicine in pediatrics. Pediatrics 122(6):1374–1386

Kemper KJ, Fletcher NB, Hamilton CA et al (2009) Impact of healing touch on pediatric oncology outpatients: pilot study. J Soc Integr Oncol 7(1):12–18

Kemper K, Drutz J, Torchia M (2012) Overview of complementary and alternative medicine in pediatrics. www.uptodate.com

Kilina AV, Kolesnikova MB (2011) [The efficacy of the application of essential oils for the prevention of acute respiratory diseases in organized groups of children], [Article in Russian]. Vestn Otorinolaringol 2011(5):51–54

Kim SY, Shin YI, Nam SO et al (2013) Concurrent Complementary and Alternative Medicine CAM and conventional rehabilitationtherapy in the management of children with developmental disorders. Evid Based Complement Alternat Med 2013(2013):812054. doi:10.1155/2013/812054. Epub 2013 Nov 12

Kligler B, Chaudhary S (2007) Peppermint oil. Am Fam Physician 75:1027–1030

Kligler B, Lee R (2004) Integrative medicine: principles for practice. The McGraw Hill Companies. New York, p 571

Kline R, Kline J, Di Palma J et al (2001) Enteric coated, pH dependent peppermimt oil capsules for the treatment of irritable bowel syndrome in children. J Pediatr 138:125–128

Kostoglou-Athanassiou I (2013) Therapeutic applications of melatonin. Ther Adv Endocrinol Metab 4(1):13–24

Kuehn BM (2009) Despite health claims by manufacturers, little oversight for homeopathic products. JAMA 302(15):1631–1634

Kulkarni A, Kaushik JS, Gupta P et al (2010) Massage and touch therapy in neonates: the current evidence. Indian Pediatr 47(9):771–776

Kumar A, Garai AK (2012) A clinical study on Pandu Roga, iron deficiency anemia, with Trikatrayadi Lauha suspension in children. J Ayurveda Integr Med 3(4):215–222. doi:10.4103/0975-9476.104446.

Kundu A, Dolan-Oves R, Dimmers M et al (2013) Reiki training for caregivers of hospitalized pediatric patient: a pilot program. Complement Ther Clin Pract 19:50–54

Kuttner L, Chambers CT, Hardial J et al (2006) A randomized trial of yoga for adolescents with irritable bowel syndrome. Pain Res Manag 11(4):217–223

Langler A, Mansky P (2012) Integrative pediatric oncology. Springer, New York, p 95

Lee AC, Kemper KJ (2000) Homeopathy and naturopathy: practice characteristics and pediatric care. Arch Pediatr Adolesc Med 154(1):75–80

Lee AC, Li DH, Kemper KJ (2000) Chiropractic care for children. Arch Pediatr Adolesc Med 154(4):401–407

Lee MS, Kim JI, Ernst E (2011) Massage therapy for children with autism spectrum disorders: a systematic review. J Clin Psychiatry 72(3):406–411

Leung B, Verhoef M (2008) Survey of parents on the use of naturopathic medicine in children-characteristics and reasons. Complement Ther Clin Pract 14(2):98–104

Lewandowski A, Ward T, Palermo T (2011) Sleep problems in children and adolescents with common medical conditions. Pediatr Clin North Am 58(3):699–713

Li JJ, Li ZW, Wang SZ et al (2011) Ningdong granule: a complementary and alternative therapy in the treatment of attention deficit/hyperactivity disorder. Psychopharmacology (Berl) 216(4):501–509

Li XM (2009) Complementary and alternative medicine in pediatric allergic disorders. Curr Opin Allergy Clin Immunol 9(2):161–167

Linde K, Barrett B, Wölkart K et al (2006) Echinacea for preventing and treating the common cold. Cochrane Database Syst Rev (1):CD000530.

Linde K, Berner MM, Kriston L (2008) St John's wort for major depression. Cochrane Database Syst Rev 4:CD000448

Lo Y (2004) What is Qi? Can we see Qi? Acupunct Today 5(9)

Loder E, Burch R, Rizzoli P (2012) The 2012 AHA/AAN guidelines for prevention of episodic migraine: a summary and comparison with other recent clinical practical guidelines. Headache 52:930–945

Lotan M (2007) Alternative therapeutic intervention for individuals with Rett syndrome. Sci World J 7:698–714

Low Dog T (2008) Smart talk on supplements and botanicals. Altern Complement 14(5):227–230

Manjunath NK, Telles S (2004) Spatial and verbal memory test scores following yoga and fine arts camp for school children. Indian J Physiol Pharmacol 48(3):353–356

Massage Therapy.com (2013) http://www.massagetherapy.com/careers/stateboards.php. Accessed 19 Dec 2013

Miele E, Pascarella F, Giannetti A et al (2009) Effect of probiotic preparation (VSL#3) on induction and maintenance of remission in children with ulcerative colitis. Am J Gastroenterol 104(2):437–434

Miller JM (2007) A study of western pharmaceuticals contained within samples of Chinese herbal/patent medicines collected from New York City's Chinatown. Legal Med 9(5):258–264

Mills MV, Henley CE, Barnes LL et al (2003) The use of osteopathic manipulative treatment as adjuvant therapy in children with recurrent acute otitis media. Arch Pediatr Adolesc Med 157(9):861–866

Moody K, Daswani D, Abrahams B et al (2009) Yoga for pain and anxiety in pediatric hematology-oncology patients: Case Series and Review of the Literature. Oral and poster presentations at the International Association of Yoga Therapists Third Annual Symposium on Yoga Therapy and Research in Los Angeles, CA. Abstract was published in the conference manual.

Moustafa Y, Kassab AN, El Sharnoubi J et al (2013) Comparative study in the management of allergic rhinitis in children using LED phototherapy and laser acupuncture. Int J Pediatr Otorhinolaryngol 77(5):658–665. doi:10.1016/j.ijporl.2013.01.006. Epub 2013 Feb 8

Muir JM (2012) Chiropractic management of a patient with symptoms of attention-deficit/hyperactivity disorder. J Chiropr Med 11(3):221–224

NAHA (2013) The national association of holistic aromatherapy. http://www.naha.org/. Accessed 17 Dec 2013

Nahin RL, Barnes PM, Stussman BJ et al (2009) Costs of Complementary and Alternative Medicine (CAM) and Frequency of Visits to CAM Practitioners: United States, 2007 National health statistics reports; no 18. Hyattsville, MD: National Center for Health Statistics.

Nam MJ, Bang YIe, Kim TI (2013) [Effects of abdominal meridian massage with aroma oils on relief of constipation among hospitalized children with brain related disabilities], [Article in Korean] J Korean Acad Nurs 43(2):247–255

National Center for Complementary and Alternative Medicine (NCCAM) National Institutes of Health, United States Department of Health and Human Services (2007) Naturopathy: An Introduction. Pub. No. D372. Accessed 25 Nov 2013

NCCAM (2013a) Traditional Chinese medicine -an introduction. http://nccam.nih.gov/health/whatiscam/chinesemed.htm. Accessed 25 Jan 2014

NCCAM-National Center for Complementary and Alternative Medicine (2013b) Acupuncture: An Introduction. Bethesda: National Center for Complementary and Alternative Medicine. NCCAM publication no. D404.

NCCAM-National Center for Complementary and Alternative Medicine (2013c) http://nccam.nih.gov/health/massage/massageintroduction.htm?nav=gsa. Accessed 19 Dec 2013

NCCAM-National Center for Complementary and Alternative Medicine (2013d) http://nccam.nih.gov/health/acupuncture/introduction.htm. Accessed 21 Jan 2014

NCCAM-National Center for Complementary and Alternative Medicine (2013e) http://nccam.nih.gov/health/reiki/introduction.htm. Accessed 4 Jan 2014

NCI (2013) Questions and answers about aromatherapy from the national cancer institute at the national institutes of health. http://www.cancer.gov/cancertopics/pdq/cam/aromatherapy/patient/Page2#Section_51. Accessed 17 Dec 2013

Ndao DH, Ladas EJ, Cheng B et al (2012) Inhalation aromatherapy in children and adolescents undergoing stem cell infusion: results of a placebo-controlled double-blind trial. Psychooncology 21(3):247–254

Nestoriuc Y, Martin A, Andrasik F (2008) Biofeedback treatment for Headache disorder: a comprehensive efficacy review. Appl Psychophysiol Biofeedback 33(3):124–140

New York Times Associated Press (2013) http://www.nytimes.com/2013/07/02/us/california-judge-allows-yoga-in-schools.html?. Accessed 8 Nov 2013

NIH Office of Dietary Supplements (2014) Fact sheet. http://ods.od.nih.gov/factsheets/Dietary-Supplements-HealthProfessional/ - Accessed 1 March 2014

Nord D, Belew J (2009) Effectiveness of the essential oils lavender and ginger in promoting children's comfort in a perianesthesia setting. J Perianesth Nurs 24(5):307–312

O'Flaherty LA, van Dijk M, Albertyn R et al (2012) Aromatherapy massage seems to enhance relaxation in children with burns: an observational pilot study. Burns 38(6):840–845

Ochi JW (2013) Acupuncture instead of codeine for tonsillectomy pain in children. Int J Pediatr Otorhinolaryngol 77(12):2058–2062. doi:10.1016/j.ijporl.2013.10.008. Epub 2013 Oct 20

Osteopathic Research Center at University of North Texas (2012) http://www.hsc.unt.edu/orc/about.html. Accessed 2 Nov 2013

Parish RA, McIntire S, Heimbach DM (1987) Garlic burns: a naturopathic remedy gone awry. Pediatr Emerg Care 3(4):258–260

Peck H, Kehle TJ, Bray MA et al (2005) Yoga as an intervention for children with attention problems. School Psychol Rev 34(3):415–424

Pepino VC, Ribeiro JD, Ribeiro MA et al (2013) Manual therapy for childhood respiratory disease: a systematic review. J Manipulative Physiol Ther 36(1):57–65

Platania-Solazzo A, Field TM, Blank J et al (1992) Relaxation therapy reduces anxiety in child and adolescent pediatric patients. Acta Paedopsychiatr 55:115–120

Pohlman KA, Holton-Brown MS (2012) Otitis media and spinal manipulative therapy: a literature review. J Chiropr Med 11(3):160–169

Posadzki P et al (2013) Osteopathic manipulative treatment for pediatric conditions: a systematic review. Pediatrics 132(1):140–152

Raghavan R, Nielson-Joseph A, Naliboff B et al (2000) The effects of yoga in adolescents with irritable bowel syndrome: A pilot study. J Adolesc Health 26:104

Rainville P, Duncan H, Price D et al (1997) Pain affect encoded in human anterior cingulate cortex but not somatosensory cortex. Science 277:968–971

Raith W, Urlesberger B, Schmölzer GM (2013) Efficacy and safety of acupuncture in preterm and term infants. Evid Based Complement Alternat Med 2013(2013):739414

Reiki (2013) International center for reiki trainig. What is reiki? http://www.reiki.org/faq/whatisreiki.html. Accessed 4 Jan 2014

Rossi E, Bartoli P, Bianchi A et al (2012) M. homeopathy in paediatric atopic diseases: long-term results in children with atopic dermatitis. Homeopathy 101(1):13–21

Rossignol D (2009) Novel and emerging treatments for autism spectrum disorders: a systematic review. Ann Clin Psychiatry 21(4):213–236

Saadat H, Kain Z (2007) Hypnosis as a therapeutic tool in pediatrics. Pediatrics 120(1):179–180

Sadler C, Vanderjagt L, Vohra S (2007) Complementary, holistic, and integrative medicine: butterbur. Pediatr Rev 28(6):235–238

Safayhi H, Sabieraj J, Sailer ER et al (1994) Chamazulene: an antioxidant-type inhibitor of leucotriene B4 formation. Planta medica 60(5):410–413

Samuel G (2008) The origins of yoga and tantra. University Press, Cambridge. ISBN 978-0-521-69534-3

Saper RB, Kales SN, Paquin J et al (2004) Heavy metal content of ayurvedic heral medicine products. JAMA 292(23):2868–2873

Saper RB, Phillips RS, Sehgal A et al (2008) Lead, mercury, and arsenic in US- and Indian-manufactured ayurvedic medicines sold via the internet. JAMA 300(8):915–923

Saps S, Seshadri R, Sztainberg M et al (2009) A prospective school-based study of abdominal pain and other common somatic complaints in children. J Pediatr 154(3):322–326

Sarrell EM, Mandelberg A, Cohen HA (2001) Efficacy of naturopathic extracts in the management of ear pain associated with acute otitis media. Arch Pediatr Adolesc Med 155(7):796–799

Sarrell EM, Cohen HA, Kahan E (2003) Naturopathic treatment for ear pain in children. Pediatrics 111(5 Pt 1):e574–579

Sarris J, Wardle J (2013) Clinical Naturopathy: An evidence-based guide to practice. 2010. Sydney: Churchill Livingstone/Elsevier Health Sciences. pp 32–36. Accessed 09 Jan 2013

Sathe K, Ali U, Ohri A (2013) Acute renal failure secondary to ingestion of ayurvedic medicine containing mercury. Indian J Nephrol 23(4):301–303. doi:10.4103/0971-4065.114485

Savic K, Pfau D, Skoric S et al (1990) The effect of Hatha yoga on poor posture in children and the psychophysiologic condition in adults. Med Pregl 43:268–272

Schwartz MS, Montgomery DD (2003) Entering the field and assuring competence. In: Schwartz MS, Andrasik F (eds) Biofeedback: a practitioner's guide, 3rd edn. The Guilford, New York

Senser S, Kelly K (2007) Complementary and alternative therapies in pediatric oncology. Pediatr Clin North Am 54(6):1046

Shafei HF, AbdelDayem SM, Mohamed NH (2012) Individualized homeopathy in a group of Egyptian asthmatic children. Homeopathy 101(4):224–230

Shah SA, Sander S, White CM et al (2007) Evaluation of Echinacea for the prevention and treatment of the common cold: a meta analysis. Lancet Infect Dis 7(7):473–480

Shamseer L, Vohra S (2009) Complementary, holistic, and integrative medicine: melatonin. Pediatr Rev 30(6):223–228

Sharma A, Gotehecha VK, Ojha NK (2012) Dyslexia: a solution through Ayurveda evidences from Ayurveda for the management of dyslexia in children: a review. Ayu 33(4):486–490

Sheldon SH (1998) Pro-convulsant effects of oral melatonin in neurologically disabled children. The Lancet 351:1254

Simeon J, Nixon MK, Jovanovic R et al (2005) Open-label pilot study of St. John's wort in adolescent depression. J Clin Adolesc Psychopharmacol 15:293–301

Soh N, Walter G (2008) Complementary medicine for psychiatric disorders in children and adolescents. Curr Opin Psychiatr 21(4):350–355

Sridharan K, Mohan R, Ramaratnam S et al (2011) Ayurvedic treatments for diabetes mellitus. Cochrane Database Syst Rev (12):CD008288. doi:10.1002/14651858.CD008288.pub2

Srivastava JK, Shankar E, Gupta S (2010) Chamomile: A herbal medicine of the past with bright future. Mol Med Rep 3(6):895–901

Stein TR, Sonty N, Saroyan JM (2012) Scratching beneath the surface: an integrative psychosocial approach to pediatric pruritus and pain. Clin Child Psychol Psychiatry 17(1):33–47

Suresh K, Pianosi P (2006) Sleep disorders in children and adolescents. BMJ 332:828–832

Suskind DL, Wahbeh G, Burpee T et al (2013) Tolerability of curcumin in pediatric inflammatory bowel disease: a forced titration study. J Pediatr Gastroenterol Nutr 56(3):277–279

Szegedi A, Kohnen R, Dienel A et al (2005) Acute treatment of moderate to severe depression with hypericum extract WS 5570 (St John's wort): a randomized controlled double blind non-inferiority trial versus paroxetine. BMJ 330(7490):503

Szymański H, Pejcz J, Jawień M et al (2006) Treatment of acute infectious diarrhoea in infants and children with a mixture of three Lactobacillus rhamnosus strains-a randomized, double-blind, placebo-controlled trial. Aliment Pharmacol Ther 23(2):247–253

Tachjian A, Maria V, Jahangir A (2010) Use of herbal products and potential interactions in patients with cardiovascular diseases. J Am Coll Cardiol 55(6):515–525

Tan G, Craine M, Blair M et al (2007) Efficacy of selected complementary and alternative medicine interventions for chronic pain. J Rehabil Res Dev 44(2):195–222

Tarnow-Mordi W, Wilkinson D, Trivedi A et al (2010) Probiotics redice all-cause mortality and necrotizing enterocolitis: it is time to change practice. Pediatrics 125(5):1068–1070

Tarsuslu T, Bol H, Simşek IE et al (2009) The effects of osteopathic treatment on constipation in children with cerebral palsy: a pilot study. J Manipulative Physiol Ther 32(8):648–653

Taylor JA, Jacobs J (2011) Homeopathic ear drops as an adjunct to standard therapy in children with acute otitis media. Homeopathy 100(3):109–115

Teixeira J (2007) Can water possibly have a memory? A skeptical view. Homeopathy 96(3):158–162

Telles S, Srinivas RB (1998) Autonomic and respiratory measures in children with impaired vision following yoga and physical activity programs. Int J Rehabil Health 4(5):117–122

Thomas DW, Greer FR (2010) American Academy of Pediatrics Committee on Nutrition; Section on Gastroenterology, Hepatology, and Nutrition. Clinical report- probiotics and prebiotics in pediatrics. Pediatrics 126(6):1217–1231

Thomas LS, Stephenson N, Swanson M et al (2013) A pilot study: the effect of healing touch on anxiety, stress, pain, pain medication usage, and physiological measures in hospitalized sickle cell disease adults experiencing a vaso-occlusive pain episode. J Holist Nurs 31(4):234–247

TTIA (2014) Therapeutic touch international association. Our definition. http://therapeutic-touch. org/. Accessed 25 Jan 2014

Uman LS, Birnie KA, Noel M et al (2013) Psychological interventions for needle-related procedural pain and distress in children and adolescents. Cochrane Database Syst Rev.10:CD005179.pub3

US Colleges of Osteopathic Medicine (2011) American Association of Colleges of Osteopathic Medicine(AACOM). Accessed 2 Nov 2013.

Valiathan MS (2006) Ayurveda: putting the house in order (pdf). Current Science. Indian Acad Sci 90(1):5–6

Valji R, Adams D, Dagenais S et al (2013) Complementary and alternative medicine: a survey of its use in pediatric oncology. Evid Based Complement Alternat Med 2013(2013):527163

Vallone SA, Miller J, Larsdotter A et al (2010) Chiropractic approach to the management of children. Chiropr Osteopat 18:16

vanderVaart S, Gijsen V, de Wildt S et al (2009) A systematic review of the therapeutic effects of Reiki. J Altern Complement Med 15(11):1157–1169

Verkamp EK, Flowers SR, Lynch-Jordan AM et al (2013) A survey of conventional and complementary therapies used by youth with juvenile-onset fibromyalgia. Pain Manag Nurs 14(4):e244–550

Wahl RA, Aldous MB, Worden KA et al (2008) Echinacea purpurea and osteopathic manipulative treatment in children with recurrent otitis media: a randomized controlled trial. BMC Complement Altern Med 8:56

Wang J (2013) Treatment of food anaphylaxis with traditional Chinese herbal remedies: from mouse model to human clinical trials. Curr Opin. Allergy Clin Immunol 13(4):386–391

Weerapong P, Hume K (2005) The mechanisms of massage and effects on performance, muscle recovery and injury prevention. Sports Med 35(3):235–256

Whitley JA, Rich BL (2008) A double-blind randomized controlled pilot trial examining the safety and efficacy of therapeutic touch in premature infants. Adv Neonatal Care 8(6):315–333

Williams TI (2006) Evaluating effects of aromatherapy massage on sleep in children with autism: a pilot study. Evid Based Complement Alternat Med 3(3):373–377

Wong J, Ghiasuddin A, Kimata C et al (2013) The impact of healing touch on pediatric oncology patients. Integr Cancer Ther 12(1):25–30

World Health Organization (2005) WHO guidelines on basic training and safety in chiropractic(PDF). ISBN 92-4-159371-7. Accessed 17 Dec 2013

Wustrow TP (2005) [Naturopathic therapy for acute otitis media. An alternative to the primary use of antibiotics], [Article in German]. HNO 53(8):728–734

Wyatt K, Edwards V, Franck L et al (2011) Cranial osteopathy for children with cerebral palsy: a randomised controlled trial. Arch Dis Child 96(6):505–512

Yang YH, Chiang BL (2013) Novel approaches to food allergy. Clin Rev Allergy Immunol 46(3):250–257

Yoga Alliance. Credentialing (2013) http://www.yogaalliance.org/Credentialing. Accessed 8 Nov 2013

Yoga for the Special Child (2013) Licensed Practitioners http://www.specialyoga.com/Licensed_ Practitioners.html. Accessed 8 Nov 2013

Yogakids (2013) http://yogakids.com/-retrieved. Accessed 8 Nov 2013

Young L, Kemper KJ (2013) Integrative care for pediatric patients with pain. J Altern Complement Med 19(7):627–632. (doi:10.1089/acm.2012.0368. Epub 2013 Feb 28)

Zhang Y, Fein EB, Fein SB (2011) Feeding of dietary botanical supplements and teas to infants in the US. Pediatrics 127(6):1060–1066

Zick S, Wright B, Sen A et al (2011) Preliminary examination of the efficacy and safety of a standardized chamomile extract for chronic primary insomnia: a randomized placebo controlled pilot study. BMC Complementary Alternative Med 11:78

Chapter 4
Current Evidence for Common Pediatric Conditions

Sanghamitra M. Misra

The Current Evidence: Allergic Rhinitis

Case Example The mother of a 15-year-old female presents with a long history of allergic rhinitis (AR). The patient has tried allergy shots but she continues to suffer. She is currently taking daily montelukast sodium and cetirizine. She wants to know more about the neti pot and potentially other nonmedicine treatments. She loves playing soccer and wants to spend more time outdoors without sneezing and rubbing her eyes.

Background Allergic rhinitis is a common, chronic medical problem that affects patients of all ages. Eighty percent of individuals develop symptoms of AR before 20 years of age, with 40 % of patients becoming symptomatic by age 6 years (Skoner 2001). Approximately 30–40 % of children suffer from AR (McCrory et al. 2003; Zutavern et al. 2008). Although allergic rhinitis is not life-threatening, it causes significant morbidity and is an economic burden.

Diagnosis The diagnosis of allergic rhinitis is made from history of typical symptoms and physical exam findings.

S. M. Misra (✉)
Academic General Pediatrics, Baylor College of Medicine, Houston, TX, USA
e-mail: smisra@bcm.edu

S. M. Misra, A. Maria Verissimo, *A Guide to Integrative Pediatrics for the Healthcare Professional,* SpringerBriefs in Public Health, DOI 10.1007/978-3-319-06835-0_4,
© Springer International Publishing Switzerland 2014

Current Evidence of Integrative Approaches to Allergic Rhinitis

Approach	Comments/Evidence
Lifestyle approaches	
Diet	Delayed solid food introduction is unlikely to affect atopic disease (Rosekranz et al. 2012)
	A more meat-based diet may pose risk for asthma and hay fever in Australian adults (Erkkola 2012)
	High maternal consumption of fruit and berry juices was positively associated with the risk of allergic rhinitis in children (Seo et al. 2013)
Environment	Environment plays a role in the onset of allergy events (Mims and Biddy 2013)
	Relocating patients to low-allergen environments demonstrates clinical improvement (AAAAI 2013a)
	Recommendations from American Academy of Allergy, Asthma and Immunology (AAAAI 2013b):
	1. Encase mattresses, box springs, and pillows in special allergen-proof fabric covers or airtight, zippered plastic covers. Bedding should be washed weekly in hot water (130° F) and dried in a hot dryer. Allergen-proof covers are available for comforters and pillows that cannot be regularly washed
	2. Keep humidity low by using a dehumidifier or air conditioning. Wall-to-wall carpeting should be removed as much as possible. Instead, throw rugs may be used if they are regularly washed or dry-cleaned
Food avoidance	Maternal dietary restriction in breastfeeding mothers to decrease risk of AR in the child is not recommended (Castro et al. 2013)
Nasal cleaning	No studies in children are available for nasal irrigation, nasal saline drops, or neti pot, but the practices cleanse the nasal passages
Probiotics	Probiotics cannot be recommended for primary prevention of atopic disease (Yao et al. 2010; Loo et al. 2013; Prescott and Tang 2005)
Vitamins	Possible benefit from vitamin C supplementation. Vitamin C intake influences AR symptoms (Ozdemir 2010)
Prevention/treatment	
Acupuncture	Penetrating needling at head acupoints is a safe therapy for patients suffering from AR, and favorable effects can be found in both the short term and long term (Wang et al. 2013)
	Acupuncture is an effective intervention that results in improved quality of life in patients with seasonal AR, but in times of limited resources for health care, acupuncture for AR may not be a cost-effective intervention (Reinhold et al. 2013)
Ayurveda	One adult study showed that Aller-7/NR-A2 (a combination of 7 herbal extracts) is well tolerated and efficacious in adult patients with allergic rhinitis (Saxena et al. 2004)
	Tinospora cordifolia (TC) significantly decreases all symptoms of allergic rhinitis in adults, and nasal smear cytology and leukocyte count correlate with clinical findings. TC is well tolerated in adults (Badar et al. 2005)
Chiropractic	No formal studies are available, but many allergy sufferers visit chiropractors before visiting otolaryngologists (Krouse and Krouse 1999)
Clinical hypnotherapy	Clinical hypnosis can lessen symptoms of AR in adults (Madrid et al. 1995)

Approach	Comments/Evidence
Herbs	Treatment with Nasya/Prevalin nasal spray was effective in adults for preventing allergic reactions induced by dust mite allergen challenge (Stoelzel et al. 2013; Kids preparation is available, but there are no available studies in children)
	Butterbur leaf special extract Ze 339 has been confirmed by 3 Good Clinical Practice trials and 2 postmarketing surveillance trials to be safe and efficacious in the treatment of adult patients with seasonal allergic rhinitis (Käufeler 2006)
	Cat's claw root is often used but needs to be used with caution in children and may interfere with effectiveness of fexofenadine (Altmedicine 2013)
	Both intranasal budesonide and oral choline are effective in relieving symptoms of allergic rhinitis in adults. Budesonide was found to be the statistically superior drug (Das et al. 2005)
	Freeze-dried nettles and a tonic made from the herb goldenseal are recommended by Mary Hardy, MD, director of integrative medicine at Cedars Sinai Medical Center in Los Angeles (WebMD 2013)
	Spirulina is clinically effective on allergic rhinitis in adults when compared with placebo (Cingi et al. 2008)
Honey	Honey ingestion at a high dose (1 g/kg body weight of honey daily in separate doses) improves the overall and individual symptoms of AR, and could serve as complementary therapy for AR (Asha'ari et al. 2013)
	Birch pollen honey could serve as complementary therapy for birch pollen allergy (Saarinen et al. 2011)
	One study in 36 adults did not confirm the widely held belief that honey relieves the symptoms of allergic rhinoconjunctivitis (Rajan et al. 2002)
Osteopathy	No available studies in children
Traditional Chinese medicine (TCM)	TCM herbs are used in addition to acupuncture for allergic rhinitis. TCM is safe and can be effective in improving symptoms (Guo and Liu 2013)
	RCM-102 (a combination of eight Chinese herbs) was safe in an adult study but not more beneficial than placebo for patients with seasonal AR (Lenon et al. 2012)
	Positive signals indicate the therapeutic effectiveness of *Astragalus membranaceus* in patients with AR (Matkovic et al. 2010)
Yoga	Per Jeff Migdow, MD, calming yoga poses can reduce stress, which in turn can improve allergic rhinitis symptoms (Migdow 2013)
	Per Harriet (Bhumi) Russell, director of Bhumi's Yoga and Wellness Center in Cleveland, Ohio, Sarvangasana (Shoulderstand) and Halasana (Plow Pose) can open nasal passages, ensuring proper drainage of sinuses, but Adho Mukha Svanasana (Downward-facing dog) and Sirsasana (Headstand) should be avoided as they can put extra pressure on nasal passages (Russell 2013)

The Current Evidence: Asthma

Case Example A 7-year-old boy with moderate, persistent asthma presents with his concerned mother. She is worried about long-term effects of inhaled steroids, and she has also heard about increase risk of sudden death associated with inhaled long-acting beta-agonists. She has come to your clinic for your opinion on alternative treatments.

Background Asthma is a chronic disease with significant morbidity and mortality. It is a complex disease with a genetic component as well as an environmental component. According to the National Heath Interview Survey, over 10 million U.S. children under age 18 (14%) have ever been diagnosed with asthma and 7 million children still have asthma (10%) (Bloom et al. 2012). A prevalence study from Canada showed that 13% of asthmatic children used CAM, and the most common forms used were vitamins, homeopathy, and acupuncture (Torres-Llenza et al. 2010).

Diagnosis The diagnosis of asthma is clinical. The most widely used classification of asthma severity is from "The Expert Panel Report 3 (EPR3): Guidelines for the Diagnosis and Management of Asthma" from the National Heart, Lung, and Blood Institute of the NIH (NHLBI 2007).

Current Evidence of Integrative Approaches to Asthma

Approach	Comments/Evidence
Lifestyle approaches	
Diet	Diet-induced weight loss can achieve significant improvements in clinical outcomes for obese children with asthma (Jensen et al. 2013)
	Consuming fruits, vegetables, and nuts (traditional Mediterranean diet) during childhood protects against asthma and rhinitis. Increased nut intake is inversely proportional to wheezing. Increased margarine intake increases risk of wheezing (Chatzi et al. 2007)
	Increased milk and egg consumption is related to decreased current wheezing (Mitchell et al. 2009)
	Benefit of omega fatty acids is controversial. Omega-6 and omega-3 fatty acids may improve allergy symptoms (Rosenlund et al. 2012). Omega-3 fatty acids may improve asthma symptoms, but omega-6 fatty acids may increase wheezing (Miles and Calder 2014). Aspirin-sensitive individuals should avoid fish oils (Jaber 2002)
	Low maternal consumption of leafy vegetables, malaceous fruits, and chocolate were positively associated with risk of wheeze in children (Erkkola et al. 2012)
	L-carnitine given at a daily dose of 1050 mg daily to children with moderate, persistent asthma showed improvement in FEV1 and overall asthma score using the Childhood Asthma Control Test (Al-Biltagi et al. 2012)

Approach	Comments/Evidence
Environment	Limit exposure to specific allergens that worsen symptoms, particularly smoke, pet dander, cockroaches, and dust (AAAAI 2013)
Food avoidance	Dairy elimination may not improve asthma symptoms (Mitchell et al. 2009)
	In a small population, dairy elimination improved respiratory tract mucus production (Bartley and McGlashan 2010)
Hydration	Limited studies have not proven importance of hydration in asthma, but hydration is important in exercise-induced asthma sufferers (Manz and Wentz 2005)
	Asthmatics who increase water consumption by 1 oz of water per kg of body weight daily have anecdotally shown improvement of symptoms (Batmanghelidj 2000)
Physical activity	Watching television for 5 or more hours per day was associated with increased risk of current wheeze (Mitchell et al. 2009)
	Sedentary lifestyle leads to excess risk of asthma during childhood (Konstantaki et al. 2013)
	Physical activity may not play an important role in the development of respiratory symptoms in preschool children (Driessen et al. 2013)
Sleep	Importance of adequate sleep was demonstrated in urban children, especially in Latino families, with asthma (Daniel et al. 2012)
Stress management	Positive results were found in asthma-related stress management training in school setting (Long et al. 2011)
	Clinical hypnosis provided improvement or resolution of pulmonary symptoms (Anbar and Hummell 2005)
Vitamin	Magnesium intake seems to have a protective effect on childhood asthma (Saadeh et al. 2013) (Rosenlund et al. 2012)
	Studies are inconclusive, but there is possible benefit of vitamin C in exercise-induced breathlessness (Milan et al. 2013)
Prevention/treatment	
Acupuncture	Acupuncture has an effect on asthma in preschool children during the treatment course as assessed by subjective parameters and need for medication (Karlson and Bennicke 2013)
	Low-intensity laser acupuncture can be a safe and effective treatment in asthmatic children (Elseify et al. 2013)
	Acupuncture has regulatory effects on immunity and may be an adjunctive therapy for allergic asthma (Yang et al. 2013)
Breathing exercises	The Papworth method (integrated breathing and relaxation exercises) appears to ameliorate respiratory symptoms, dysfunctional breathing, and adverse mood in adults compared with usual care (Holloway and West 2007)
	The Buteyko method (used by millions in the former Soviet Union) teaches breathing exercises through an instructional VDO to increase $PaCO_2$. The method showed significant improvement in quality of life and reduction of bronchodilator use in a study of 36 patients (Opat et al. 2000)
Chiropractic	There has been a favorable response to subjective and objective outcome measures of asthma in both patients and parents to spinal manipulative therapy (SMT) (Gleberzon et al. 2012)

Approach	Comments/Evidence
Herbs/Ayurveda/ traditional Chinese medicine	One study in adults showed *Boswellia serrata*, *Curcuma longa*, and Glycyrrhiza have pronounced effects in the management of bronchial asthma (Houssen et al. 2010)
	In studies of Bharangyadi Avaleha and Vasa Avaleha, results have shown less recurrence of asthma symptoms (Gohel et al. 2011)
	In a systematic review, "Single studies of Boswellia, Mai-Men-Dong-Tang, Pycnogenol, Jia-Wei-Si-Jun-Zi-Tang and *Tylophora indica* showed potential to improve lung function, and a study of 1.8-Cineol (eucalyptol) showed reduced daily oral steroid dosage" (Clark et al. 2010)
Osteopathy	Benefits not proven in systematic studies, but small studies show benefit (Posadzki et al. 2013)
Yoga	There have been positive associations shown between exercise habit after school and muscular strength and endurance among asthmatic children (Chen et al. 2009)
	There is significant benefit of yoga seen soon after starting the exercise (Khanam et al. 1996)
	Physiological benefits of yoga for the pediatric population may help children through the rehabilitation process (Galantino et al. 2008)

The Current Evidence: Attention-Deficit/Hyperactivity Disorder

Case Example A 9-year-old male presents to your clinic with a history of attention-deficit/hyperactivity disorder (ADHD), inattentive-type. He has been on Adderall and Vyvanse over the last 2 years, and his mother is concerned that he is losing weight due to poor appetite. The pediatrician thinks that the child will not succeed in school without stimulant medication.

Background ADHD is a commonly diagnosed childhood disorder characterized by impulsivity, inattention, and hyperactivity. ADHD affects up to 10 % of children in the United States. Many different forms of CAM are used for ADHD but treatments appear to be most effective when prescribed holistically and according to each individual's characteristic symptoms (Pellow et al. 2011).

Diagnosis ADHD is diagnosed according to the American Psychiatric Association's Diagnostic and Statistical Manual of Mental Disorders—Fifth Edition (DSM-5). The DSM-5 has defined consensus criteria for the diagnosis of ADHD, which is categorized into three divisions: 1) Predominantly hyperactive, 2) Predominantly impulsive, and 3) Combined (APA 2013).

Current Evidence for Integrative Approaches to ADHD

Approach	Comments/Evidence
Lifestyle approaches	
Diet	From a 2013 editorial by Rommelse and Buitelaar, "...there is a future for dietary interventions in ADHD clinical practice, but valid and important points of criticism should be tackled first before implementation in clinical practice can be considered" (Rommelse and Buitelaar 2013)
Food avoidance	Salicylate elimination diet: not enough evidence to recommend (Gray et al. 2013)
	Artificial food color (AFC): A trial of AFC elimination is appropriate in cases where a child has not responded satisfactorily to conventional treatment or whose parents wish to pursue a dietary investigation. Oligoantigenic diet studies suggested that some children, in addition to being sensitive to AFCs, are also sensitive to common nonsalicylate foods (milk, chocolate, soy, eggs, wheat, corn, legumes) as well as salicylate-containing grapes, tomatoes, and oranges. Trial of elimination may be satisfactory (Stevens et al. 2011)
	Free fatty acid supplementation produces small but significant reductions in ADHD symptoms. AFC exclusion can be beneficial in individuals with food sensitivities. Better evidence for efficacy from blinded assessments is required for behavioral interventions, neurofeedback, cognitive training, and restricted elimination diets before they can be supported as treatments for core ADHD symptoms (Sonuga-Barke et al. 2013)
	The large Impact of Nutrition on Children with ADHD (INCA) study stated, "A strictly supervised restricted elimination diet is a valuable instrument to assess whether ADHD is induced by food. The prescription of diets on the basis of IgG blood tests should be discouraged" (Pelsser et al. 2011)
Vitamins	One study showed that lower maternal folate level in early pregnancy might impair fetal brain development and affect hyperactivity/inattention and peer problems in childhood (Schlotz et al. 2010)
	Mineral supplementation is indicated for those with documented deficiencies (iron, zinc) but is not supported for others with ADHD (Hurt et al. 2011; Sarris et al. 2011)
	Carnitine/l-acetyl carnitine supplementation may benefit symptom of inattention, but evidence is limited and inconclusive (Hurt et al. 2011; Abbasi et al. 2011)
	There is inconclusive evidence for use of omega-3 (Sarris et al. 2011)
Physical activity	Physical exercise may lessen severity of children's ADHD symptoms (Rommel et al. 2013)
Environment	Doubling the prenatal lead exposure (cord blood lead levels) was associated with a 3.43 times higher risk for hyperactivity in both boys and girls (Sioen et al. 2013)
	Postnatal lead exposure may be associated with higher risk of clinical ADHD, but not the postnatal exposure to mercury or cadmium (Kim et al. 2013)

Approach	Comments/Evidence
Treatment	
Yoga	Yoga has shown promise as an add-on therapy for ADHD (Hariprasad et al. 2013)
Meditation	In a 2010 Cochrane database survey, the authors were unable to draw any conclusions regarding the effectiveness of meditation therapy for ADHD (Krisanaprakornkit et al. 2010)
Yoga/meditation/play therapy	The "Climb-Up" program in India enlisted 69 children with ADHD and instituted peer-mediated in-school yoga, meditation, and play therapy twice weekly. This resulted in remarkable improvements in the students' school performances that were sustained throughout the year (Mehta et al. 2011; Mehta et al. 2012)
Osteopathy	No studies available
Herbals/traditional Chinese medicine	*Pinus marinus* (French maritime pine bark) and a Chinese herbal formula (Ningdong) were found to have moderate evidence in a systematic review that also showed that *Ginkgo biloba* (ginkgo) and *Hypercium perforatum* (St. John's wort) are ineffective in treating ADHD (Hurt et al. 2011)
	Compound herbal preparation (CHP): Under the brand name Nurture & Clarity, the combination of *Paeoniae alba, Withania somnifera, Centella asiatica, Spirulina platensis, Bacopa monieri,* and *Mellissa officinalis* demonstrated improved attention, cognition, and impulse control, indicating promise as an ADHD treatment in children (Katz et al. 2010)
Naturopathy	No studies available
Chiropractic	A case study in a 5-year-old showed benefit of chiropractic care, including spinal manipulative therapy and soft tissue therapy, for ADHD symptoms (Muir 2012)
	There are measurable benefits of chiropractic spinal manipulative therapy for children with ADHD (Alcantara and Davis 2010)
Homeopathy	In a systematic review from 2011, there was insufficient evidence to draw robust conclusions about the effectiveness of any particular form of homeopathy for the treatment of ADHD (Keen and Hadijikoumi 2011)
	Another review in 2011 concluded: "The database on studies of homeopathy and placebo in psychiatry (including ADHD) is very limited, but results do not preclude the possibility of some benefit (Davidson et al. 2011)
Ayurveda	An ayurvedic compound drug and Shirodhara were both effective in improving the reaction time of ADHD-affected children (Singhal et al. 2010)
Acupuncture	There is limited data on the effectiveness of acupuncture as a treatment for ADHD (Lee et al. 2011; Li et al. 2011)

The Current Evidence: Migraine Headaches

Case Example A 13-year-old female presents with a 5-year history of migraine headaches. She has consulted with a pediatric neurologist and had a reportedly negative work-up for concerning pathology. The neurologist placed the patient on propranolol for migraine prophylaxis, and she uses ibuprofen for abortive therapy. Her mother is concerned about long-term side effects of propranolol, and is curious about alternative treatments.

Background Headache is one of the most common neurological symptoms reported in childhood and adolescence, leading to high levels of school absences and being associated with several comorbid conditions including depression, anxiety disorders, epilepsy, sleep disorders, ADHD, and Tourette syndrome. It has also been shown to be associated with atopic disease and cardiovascular disease, especially ischemic stroke and patent foramen ovale (PFO) (Bellini et al. 2013).

Diagnosis The International Headache Society has established diagnostic criteria for migraine headaches in children and adolescents (ISH 2004).

Current Evidence Behind Integrative Approaches to Migraine Headaches

Approach	Comments/Evidence
Lifestyle approaches	
Diet	Three meals and one to two snacks per day should be eaten at routine times
	Breakfast should not be skipped
Hydration	Inadequate hydration should be avoided. Adolescents are encouraged to drink 2 liters of noncaffeinated liquids, ideally water, per day, increasing to 3 L a day during the summer and periods of exertion (Lewis et al. 2005)
Food avoidance	Avoidance diets are not recommended unless a trigger has been identified (Millichap and Yee 2003). Common triggers include chocolate, citrus fruits, cheeses, processed meats, yogurt, fried foods, monosodium glutamate, aspartame, alcoholic beverages, and caffeine
Physical activity	At least 30 min of enjoyable, aerobic activity should be performed 3–7 days a week with family or friends. Migraine sufferers and their parents should AVOID excessive or unrealistic expectations of performance in school, athletics, and other activities which may contribute to migraines (Holroyd et al. 1991; Ahn 2013; Gil-Martinez et al. 2013)
Stress management	Yoga and meditation are beneficial (John et al. 2007)
Sleep	Adequate nightly sleep is essential and good sleep hygiene is important (Lewis et al. 2005)
	According to Bigal and Hargreaves, "The relationship between sleep and migraine headaches is complex. Changes in sleep patterns can trigger migraine attacks, and sleep disorders may be associated with increased migraine frequency" (Bigal and Hargreaves 2013)

Approach	Comments/Evidence
Prevention/Prophylaxis	
Butterbur (Petasites)	AHS/AAN Migraine Prevention Guidelines 2012 label Butterbur as Level A (effective)
	Adults: 50–75 mg BID (Loder et al. 2012)
	Dosing from a study in children ages 6–17 years was 50–150 mg of butterbur root extract daily (Pothman and Danesch 2005)
Feverfew (*Tanacetum parthenium*)	AHS/AAN Migraine Prevention Guidelines 2012 label Feverfew as Level B (probably effective) (Loder et al. 2012)
	Adults: 50–300 mg BID; 2.08–18.75 mg TID for MIG-99 preparation
Coenzyme Q10	Numerous studies have shown efficacy (Hershey et al. 2007; Slater et al. 2011)
	AHS/AAN Migraine Prevention Guidelines 2012 label Coenzyme Q10 as Level C (possibly effective)
	Adults: 100 mg TID (Loder et al. 2012)
Magnesium	Studied in children ages 3–17 years (9 mg/kg per day by mouth divided 3 times a day with food) (Wang et al. 2003)
Acupuncture	Acupuncture is effective and should be considered as a prophylactic measure for patients with frequent or insufficiently controlled migraine attacks (Schiapparelli et al. 2010)
	According to a Cochrane review of studies in adults by Linde and colleagues, "Acupuncture is at least as effective, or possibly more effective than, prophylactic drug treatment, and has fewer adverse effects"(Linde et al. 2009)
Mind-body Therapies	Biofeedback, Clinical Hypnosis, and Progressive Relaxation can improve migraines (Nestoriuc and Martin 2007; Legarda et al. 2011; Shah and Kalra 2009; Fentress et al. 1986)
Music Therapy	Music therapy is a possible treatment for schoolchildren (Oelkers-Ax et al. 2008)
Treatment/Abortive	
Feverfew/Ginger	Sublingual feverfew/ginger appears safe and effective as a first-line abortive treatment for those who frequently experience mild headache prior to the onset of moderate to severe headache (Cady et al. 2011)
Ginger (*Zingiber officinale*)	The effectiveness of ginger powder in the treatment of common migraine attacks is statistically comparable to sumatriptan (Mehdi et al. 2013
	Ginger is considered to be generally safe by the FDA
Migrelief (Feverfew + B2 + Magnesium)	A children's formulation is available
	No specific studies are available in children
Capsaicin	For children, recommend in food (Kemper 1996)
Intravenous Magnesium	30 mg/kg with a maximum dose of 2000 mg infused over 30 min (Gertsch et al. 2014)

The Current Evidence: Otalgia and Otitis Media

Case Example The mother of a 2-year-old daughter brings in her child for 1-day history of right-sided ear pain. Mom is concerned about the possibility of an ear infection and has read about the consequences of antibiotic overuse. She wants to take a holistic approach to her child's ear pain. The child has not had fever or any other symptoms. This is the child's first episode of ear pain. She was breastfed for 18 months and is up to date on her immunizations.

Background Ear pain, effusions, and infections are frequent reasons for physician office visits. The correct differentiation of otalgia versus serous otitis media versus purulent otitis media is vital to the appropriate treatment of an ear (Wald 2005). A study from Italy in 2011 showed that 46 % of the children used complementary and alternative medicine (CAM) for recurrent acute otitis media (AOM), significantly more than the number who used immunizations for influenza or pneumococcus. The main reasons for using CAM were a fear of the adverse effects of conventional medicine (40 %) and to increase host defenses (20 %). CAM was widely seen as safe (95 %) and highly effective (68 %) (Marchisio et al. 2011).

Diagnosis The American Academy of Pediatrics in 2013 published an updated "Clinical Practice Guideline: The Diagnosis and Management of Acute Otitis Media" which provides a specific, stringent definition of AOM, addresses pain management and initial observation versus antibiotic treatment, provides appropriate choices of antibiotic agents and preventive measures, and describes management of recurrent AOM (Lieberthal et al. 2013).

Current Evidence of Integrative Approaches to Otalgia and Otitis Media

Approach	Comments/Evidence
Lifestyle approaches	
Diet	A diet high in fruits and vegetables may be protective against AOM (Esplugues et al. 2013)
Environment	Removal of second-hand smoke is protective (Strachan and Cook 1998; Uhari et al. 1996; Ladomenou et al. 2010)
Food Avoidance	Stop bottle and pacifier use after 1 year of age (Uhari et al. 1996; Ladomenou et al. 2010)
Physical Activity	Baby swimming (infants <6 months of age) does not increase risk of AOM (Nystad et al. 2008)
	According to Wang et al, "Patients with chronic otitis media with active drainage should avoid swimming.... Children with ventilation tubes may surface swim in clean, chlorinated swimming pool" (Wang et al. 2005)
Vitamins and Supplements	Zinc and vitamin A deficiency may lead to middle ear disease (Elemraid et al. 2009)
	Vitamin A deficiency has been shown as a significant factor in the etiology of acute and chronic suppurative otitis media (Lasisi 2009)
	The level of Vitamin 25(OH)D needed to prevent ear infections has not been defined (Linday et al. 2008)
	One study showed decreased antibiotic usage in children given cod liver oil (long chain omega-3 fatty acid) and selenium supplementation (Linday et al. 2002)

Approach	Comments/Evidence
Prevention/Treatment	
Chiropractic	There is limited quality evidence for use of spinal manipulative therapy in children with AOM (Pohlman and Holton-Brown 2012).
Herbals	Herbal eardrops may help relieve symptoms (Levi et al. 2013)
	Echinacea purpurea may increase risk of AOM when used for upper respiratory infections (Wahl et al. 2008)
	Xylitol gum, syrup, and lozenges have shown efficacy in the treatment of acute otitis media (Blazek-O'Neill 2005)
	No studies are available on common herbs used for ear pain including peppermint oil, cloves oil or calendula oil, olive oil, garlic cloves in mustard oil, Mullein flower oil, holy basil leaves juice, and lemon balm
Homeopathy	Using homeopathy may decrease antibiotic usage (Fixsen 2013)
	Homeopathy may help decrease pain and lead to faster resolution of infection (Levi et al. 2013)
Naturopathy	Otikon is as effective as anaesthetic ear drops and appropriate for management of AOM-associated ear pain (Sarrell et al. 2001; Sarrell et al. 2003).
Osteopathy	Not enough evidence exists to make a recommendation (Posadzki et al. 2013; Wahl et al. 2008)

The Current Evidence: Upper Respiratory Tract Infections

Clinical Case A 12-year-old male presents because of a history of recurrent upper respiratory tract infections (URIs). His mother is concerned that his pediatrician is always prescribing antibiotics, and she is very worried about overusage of antibiotics. She wants to try a more holistic approach to her child's health. She has tried giving the child Echinacea for prevention of URIs but had to stop the herb due to the side effect of headaches. The mother is open to any suggestions.

Background The common cold is the most common illness in pediatrics. Infants and children generally have prolonged symptoms compared to adults. This often leads to parents feeling helpless, especially since allopathy prescribes supportive care with little intervention for URIs. The common cold causes school absenteeism and in turn caregiver work absenteeism. In the US, the estimated economic yearly cost of lost productivity due to the common cold approaches $ 25 billion, of which $ 8 billion is attributed to absenteeism, and $ 230 million is attributed to caregiver absenteeism (Bramley et al. 2002).

Diagnosis A common cold is diagnosed by the confluence of common URI symptoms (sore throat, runny nose, sneezing, coughing, fever, and headache) and their duration.

Integrative Approaches to Upper Respiratory Tract Infections

Approach	Comments/Evidence
Lifestyle approaches	
Diet	No studies are available on the role of diet in upper respiratory infections in children
Physical Activity	Vigorous physical activity has a significant association with symptoms of eczema, but not rhinoconjunctivitis (Mitchell et al. 2013)
Vitamins	Vitamin A and iron supplementation together may decrease symptoms of runny nose, fever, and cough (Chen et al. 2013)
	Lower serum vitamin 25(OH)D levels were associated with increased risk of laboratory-confirmed viral URI in children from Canadian Hutterite communities (Science et al. 2013)
	A systematic review and meta-analysis in 2012 concluded that vitamin D supplementation decreases the events related to respiratory tract infections; however, there is a need for more well-conducted clinical trials to confirm this conclusion (Charan et al. 2012)
	A review study by Esposito et al. in 2013 concluded that "further studies are needed to evaluate the impact of vitamin D deficiency and insufficiency in terms of the epidemiology and outcomes of pediatric respiratory tract infection, and whether VitD supplementation favours a positive outcome" (Esposito et al. 2013)
	With vitamin C supplementation, duration of colds was reduced by 14 % in children (7–21 %), and 1–2 g/day of vitamin C given to children shortened colds by 18 %. Given the consistent effect of vitamin C on the duration and severity of colds in supplementation studies, and the low cost and safety, it may be a useful adjunct for common cold patients (Hemilä and Chalker 2013)
	In a cluster-randomized study of pediatric visits for upper respiratory illness during the winter and early spring, cod liver oil with a multivitamin containing selenium decreased mean visits/subject/month by 36–58 % (Linday 2010)
	Zinc sulfate improves symptoms in children (Fashner et al. 2012)
Prevention/Treatment	
Chiropractic	The use of manual techniques on children with respiratory diseases may have benefit. Chiropractic, osteopathic medicine, and massage are the most common interventions. The lack of standardized procedures and a limited variety of methods used evidenced the need for more studies on the subject (Pepino et al. 2013)

Approach	Comments/Evidence
Herbals	Echinacea is ineffective in children (Di Pierro et al. 2012)
	Echinacea purpurea may be effective in reducing the occurrence of subsequent URIs in children (Weber et al. 2005)
	Polinacea (a highly standardized form of echinacea) could be used for improving the immune response to influenza vaccine (Di Pierro et al. 2012)
	Pelargonium sidoides (geranium) extract and buckwheat honey improve symptoms in children (Linday 2010)
	Prophylactic probiotics and the herbal preparation Chizukit reduce the incidence of colds in children (Fashner et al. 2012)
	Elderberry extract (Sambucol) may be useful for the treatment of viral influenza infections (Vlachojannis et al. 2010)
	A systematic review concluded that North American ginseng appears to be effective in shortening the duration of colds or URIs in healthy adults when taken preventively for durations of 8–16 weeks (Seida et al. 2011)
	Standard doses of ginseng were well tolerated in children in a randomized, controlled trial of 2 dosing schedules (Vohra et al. 2008)
	Astragalus membranaceus supplementation resulted in strongest activation and proliferation of immune cells in a small double-blind, placebo-controlled study that also included Echinacea purpurea and Glycyrrhiza glabra (Brush et al. 2006)
Homeopathy	A pilot study in children concluded that utility of the homeopathic remedies prescribed is based on the concept of individualization in the treatment of URIs in children (Ramchandani 2010)
	There is insufficient good evidence in adults to enable robust conclusions about Oscillococcinum in the prevention or treatment of influenza and influenza-like illness (Mathie et al. 2012)
Massage Therapy	Massage has proved very helpful in improving general constitution, enhancing the immune functions, and preventing and treating URIs (Zhu et al. 1998)

The Current Evidence: Weight Loss

Case Example A 16-year-old overweight female comes for her annual check-up. During the HEADS exam when the mother has stepped out of the room, she asks about weight loss drugs. Her friend has lost 10 pounds in 2 months by crushing birdseeds and drinking a tea made from the seeds. She wants to know if she should drink the tea or if you have any other suggestions on weight loss remedies.

Background Obesity is a common problem in childhood and adolescents. According to Ogden et al, "in 2009–2010, the prevalence of obesity in children and adolescents was 16.9 %" (Ogden et al. 2012).

Diagnosis The body mass index (BMI) is the accepted standard measure of overweight and obesity for children 2 years of age and older (Deurenberg et al. 1991). All pediatric healthcare professionals should be screening for and guiding the prevention and treatment of normoweight, overweight and obese patients.

Current Evidence for Integrative Approaches to Weight Loss

Approach	Comments/Evidence
Lifestyle approaches	
Diet	Two of the many available resources:
	1. American Academy of Pediatrics–Texas Pediatric Society Obesity Toolkit (TPS 2013)
	2. Academy of Nutrition and Dietetics (Hoelscher et al. 2013)
	According to Ho et al., "In the short to medium term, a prescriptive dietary intervention approach is a well-accepted and suitable option for obese adolescents with clinical features of insulin resistance. It may reduce external and emotional eating, led to modest weight loss and did not cause any adverse effect on dietary restraint" (Ho et al. 2013)
Food Avoidance	Benefit from decreased consumption of sugar-sweetened beverages (Malik et al. 2013; Ebbeling et al. 2012)
	Possible benefit from decreased salt intake (Grimes et al. 2013a)
Vitamins	Vitamin D: The correction of poor vitamin D status through dietary supplementation may be an effective addition to the standard treatment of obesity and its associated insulin resistance (Belenchia et al. 2013). Overweight/obese and non-Hispanic black children are especially likely to be at risk for inadequate 25OHD when not consuming the recommended daily allowance (Au et al. 2013)
	100% Fruit juice in moderation may improve nutrient intake and likely does not lead to overweight/obesity (O'Neil et al. 2010, 2012; Nicklas et al. 2008)
Physical Activity	A model of exercise prescription (supervised play-based physical activity) could be considered world-wide by clinicians to improve fitness base in adolescents and help to combat the growing epidemic of childhood obesity (Meucci et al. 2013)
	The overall effectiveness of video games that include exercise has not been well studied
Sleep	A good night's sleep seems essential to good health, but the relationship between sleep and obesity in children has not been determined. One study has shown that sleep duration does not predict obesity up to age 6–7 years (Hiscock et al. 2011)
Environment	Reduce exposure to BPA. Urinary BPA concentration has been associated with obesity in children and adolescents. Explanations of the association cannot rule out the possibility that obese children ingest food with higher BPA content or have greater adipose stores of BPA (Trasande et al. 2012)
Prevention/Treatment	
Acupuncture	Acupuncture therapy significantly reduces BMI and abdominal adipose tissue in obese children (Zhang et al. 2011)
	A study in adults showed that acupuncture therapy can reduce body weight by accelerating the peristalsis and inhibiting the hunger sensation (Wang et al. 2007). Photo-acupuncture is a safe, painless, nontraumatic, and effective method for treatment of obesity that is easily accepted by children (Yu et al. 1998)
	Acupuncture should be recommended for comprehensive treatment of children with constitutional exogenic obesity (Gadzhiev et al. 1993)

Approach	Comments/Evidence
Ayurveda	A number of ayurvedic drugs have hypolipidemic and anti-obesity/hypoglycemic properties (Kumari et al. 2013)
	Shilajatu (Asphaltum) processed with Agnimantha (Clerodendrum phlomidis Linn.) is statistically effective in helping adults with obesity (Pattonder et al. 2011)
Chiropractic	No available studies in children
Clinical Hypnosis	Adult studies show benefit for weight loss (Steyer and Ables 2009)
	No available studies in children
Herbals	Although not studied in children, foods containing diacylglycerol oil promote weight loss and body fat reduction and may be useful as an adjunct to diet therapy in the management of obesity (Maki et al. 2002)
	A case study showed seizures from caffeine in a weight loss herbal product named Zantrex-3 that included niacin, caffeine, and numerous herbs (Pendleton et al. 2012)
	In a systematic review of adults from 2009, compounds containing ephedra, Cissus quadrangularis (CQ), ginseng, bitter melon, and zingiber were found to be effective in the management of obesity. No significant adverse effects or mortality were observed except in studies with supplements containing ephedra, caffeine, and Bofutsushosan (Hasani-Ranjbar et al. 2009)
	Green tea extract for weight loss is a potential cause of acute liver failure (Patel et al. 2013)
Homeopathy	There are no available studies in children
	One adult review stated that there is not enough evidence to recommend homeopathy for weight loss (Pittler and Ernst 2005)

References

AAAAI (2013a) Indoor allergens: tips to remember. http://www.aaaai.org/conditions-and-treatments/library/at-a-glance/indoor-allergens.aspx. Accessed 26 Dec 2013

AAAAI (2013b) The American Academy of Allergy, Asthma and Immunology. https://www.aaaai.org/conditions-and-treatments/library/at-a-glance/prevention-of-allergies-and-asthma-in-children.aspx. Accessed 28 Dec 2013

Abbasi SH, Heidari S, Mohammadi MR et al (2011) Acetyl-L-carnitine as an adjunctive therapy in the treatment of attention-deficit/hyperactivity disorder in children and adolescents: a placebo-controlled trial. Child Psychiatry Hum Dev 42(3):367–375

Ahn AH (2013) Why does increased exercise decrease migraine? Curr Pain Headache Rep 17(12):379

Al-Biltagi M, Isa M, Bediwy AS et al (2012) L-carnitine improves the asthma control in children with moderate persistent asthma. J Allergy (Cairo) 2012:509730. doi:10.1155/2012/509730. (Epub 2011 Nov 23)

Alcantara J, Davis J (2010) The chiropractic care of children with attention-deficit/hyperactivity disorder: a retrospective case series. Explore (NY) 6(3):173–182

Altmedicine (2013) What is cat's claw? http://altmedicine.about.com/od/herbsupplementguide/a/Cats_Claw.htm. Accessed 27 Dec 2013

Anbar RD, Hummell KE (2005) Teamwork approach to clinical hypnosis at a pediatric pulmonary center. Am J Clin Hypn 48(1):45–49

APA—American Psychiatric Association (2013) Attention-deficit/hyperactivity disorder. In: American Psychiatric Association (ed) Diagnostic and statistical manual of mental disorders, 5th edn. Amer Psychiatric, Arlington, p 59

Asha'ari ZA, Ahmad MZ, Jihan WS et al (2013) Ingestion of honey improves the symptoms of allergic rhinitis: evidence from a randomized placebo-controlled trial in the east coast of Peninsular Malaysia. Ann Saudi Med 33(5):469–475

Au LE, Rogers GT, Harris SS et al (2013) Associations of vitamin D intake with 25-hydroxyvitamin D in overweight and racially/ethnically diverse US children. J Acad Nutr Diet 113(11):1511–1516

Badar VA, Thawani VR, Wakode PT et al (2005) Efficacy of *Tinospora cordifolia* in allergic rhinitis. J Ethnopharmacol 96(3):445–449

Bartley J, McGlashan SR (2010) Does milk increase mucus production? Med Hypotheses 74(4):732–734

Batmanghelidj F (2000) ABC of asthma, allergies and Lupus-eradicate asthma-now! Global Health Solutions, Melbourne

Belenchia AM, Tosh AK, Hillman LS et al (2013) Correcting vitamin D insufficiency improves insulin sensitivity in obese adolescents: a randomized controlled trial. Am J Clin Nutr 97(4):774–781

Bellini B, Arruda M, Cescut A et al (2013) Headache and comorbidity in children and adolescents. J Headache Pain 14(1):79

Bigal ME, Hargreaves RJ (2013) Why does sleep stop migraine? Curr Pain Headache Rep 17(10):369

Blazek-O'Neill B (2005) Complementary and alternative medicine in allergy, otitis media, and asthma. Curr Allergy Asthma Rep 5(4):313–318

Bloom B, Cohen RA, Freeman G (2012) 2011 summary health statistics for U.S. children: National Health Interview Survey, National Center for Health Statistics. Vital Health Stat 10(250):1–80

Bramley TJ, Lerner D, Sames M (2002) Productivity losses related to the common cold. J Occup Environ Med 44(9):822

Brush J, Mendenhall E, Guggenheim A et al (2006) The effect of *Echinacea purpurea*, *Astragalus membranaceus* and *Glycyrrhiza glabra* on CD69 expression and immune cell activation in humans. Phytother Res 20(8):687–695

Cady RK, Goldstein J, Nett R et al (2011) A double-blind placebo-controlled pilot study of sublingual feverfew and ginger (LipiGesic™ M) in the treatment of migraine. Headache 51(7):1078–1086

Castro TM, Marinho DR, Cavalcante CC (2013) The impact of environmental factors on quality of life and symptoms of children with allergic rhinitis. Braz J Otorhinolaryngol 79(5):569–574

Charan J, Goyal JP, Saxena D et al (2012) Vitamin D for prevention of respiratory tract infections: a systematic review and meta-analysis. Pharmacol Pharmacother 3(4):300–303

Chatzi L, Apostolaki G, Bibakis I et al (2007) Protective effect of fruits, vegetables and the Mediterranean diet on asthma and allergies among children in Crete. Thorax 62(8):677–683

Chen TL, Mao HC, Lai CH et al (2009) The effect of yoga exercise intervention on health related physical fitness in school-age asthmatic children. Hu Li Za Zhi 56(2):42–52. (Article in Chinese)

Chen K, Chen XR, Zhang L et al (2013) Effect of simultaneous supplementation of vitamin A and iron on diarrheal and respiratory tract infection in preschool children in Chengdu City, China. Nutrition 29(10):1197–1203

Cingi C, Conk-Dalay M, Cakli H et al (2008) The effects of spirulina on allergic rhinitis. Eur Arch Otorhinolaryngol 265(10):1219–23

Clark CE, Arnold E, Lasserson TJ et al (2010) Herbal interventions for chronic asthma in adults and children: a systematic review and meta-analysis. Prim Care Respir J 19(4):307–314

Daniel LC, Boergers J, Kopel SJ et al (2012) Missed sleep and asthma morbidity in urban children. Ann Allergy Asthma Immunol 109(1):41–46

Das S, Gupta K, Gupta A et al (2005) Comparison of the efficacy of inhaled budesonide and oral choline in patients with allergic rhinitis. Saudi Med J 26(3):421–424

Davidson JR, Crawford C, Ives JA et al (2011) Homeopathic treatments in psychiatry: a systematic review of randomized placebo-controlled studies. J Clin Psychiatry 72(6):795–805

Deurenberg P, Weststrate JA, Seidell JC (1991) Body mass index as a measure of body fatness: age- and sex-specific prediction formulas. Br J Nutr 65(2):105

Di Pierro F, Rapacioli G, Ferrara T et al (2012) Use of a standardized extract from *Echinacea angustifolia* (Polinacea) for the prevention of respiratory tract infections. Altern Med Rev 17(1):36–41

Driessen LM, Kiefte-de Jong JC, Jaddoe VW et al (2013) Physical activity and respiratory symptoms in children: the generation R study. Pediatr Pulmonol 49:36–42

Ebbeling CB, Feldman HA, Chomitz VR et al (2012) Randomized trial of sugar-sweetened beverages and adolescent body weight. N Engl J Med 367(15):1407

Elemraid MA, Mackenzie IJ, Fraser WD et al (2009) Nutritional factors in the pathogenesis of ear disease in children: a systematic review. Ann Trop Paediatr 29(2):85–99

Elseify MY, Mohammed NH, Alsharkawy AA et al (2013) Laser acupuncture in treatment of childhood bronchial asthma. J Complement Integr Med 10(1):199–203

Erkkola M, Nwaru BI, Kaila M et al (2012) Risk of asthma and allergic outcomes in the offspring in relation to maternal food consumption during pregnancy: a Finnish birth cohort study. Pediatr Allergy Immunol 23(2):186–194

Esplugues A, Estarlich M, Sunyer J et al (2013) Prenatal exposure to cooking gas and respiratory health in infants is modified by tobacco smoke exposure and diet in the INMA birth cohort study. Environ Health 12(1):100

Esposito S, Baggi E, Bianchini S et al (2013) Role of vitamin D in children with respiratory tract infection. Int J Immunopathol Pharmacol 26(1):1–13

Fashner J, Ericson K, Werner S (2012) Treatment of the common cold in children and adults. Am Fam Physician 86(2):153–159

Fentress DW, Masek BJ, Mehegan JE et al (1986) Biofeedback and relaxation-response training in the treatment of pediatric migraine. Dev Med Child Neurol 28(2):139

Fixsen A (2013) Should homeopathy be considered as part of a treatment strategy for otitis media with effusion in children? Homeopathy 102(2):145–150

Gadzhiev AA, Mugarab-Samedi VV, Isaev II et al (1993) Acupuncture therapy of constitution-exogenous obesity in children. Probl Endokrinol (Mosk) 39(3):21–24. (Article in Russian)

Galantino ML, Galbavy R, Quinn L (2008) Therapeutic effects of yoga for children: a systematic review of the literature. Pediatr Phys Ther 20(1):66–80

Gertsch E, Loharuka S, Wolter-Warmerdam K et al (2014) Intravenous magnesium as acute treatment for headaches: a pediatric case series. J Emerg Med 46:308–312. (pii: S0736–4679(13) 01019–6)

Gil-Martinez A, Kindelan-Calvo P, Agudo-Carmona D et al (2013) Therapeutic exercise as treatment for migraine and tension-type headaches: a systematic review of randomised clinical trials. Rev Neurol 57(10):433–443

Gleberzon BJ, Arts J, Mei A et al (2012) The use of spinal manipulative therapy for pediatric health conditions: a systematic review of the literature. J Can Chiropr Assoc 56(2):128–141

Gohel SD, Anand IP, Patel KS (2011) A comparative study on efficacy of Bharangyadi Avaleha and Vasa Avaleha in the management of Tamaka Shwasa with reference to childhood asthma. Ayu 32(1):82–89

Gray PE, Mehr S, Katelaris CH et al (2013) Salicylate elimination diets in children: is food restriction supported by the evidence? Med J Aust 198(11):600–602

Grimes CA, Riddell LJ, Campbell KJ, Nowson CA (2013a) Dietary salt intake, sugar-sweetened beverage consumption, and obesity risk. Pediatrics 131(1):14–21

Guo H, Liu MP (2013) Mechanism of traditional Chinese medicine in the treatment of allergic rhinitis. Chin Med J (Engl) 126(4):756–760

Hariprasad VR, Arasappa R, Varambally S et al (2013) Feasibility and efficacy of yoga as an add-on intervention in attention deficit-hyperactivity disorder: an exploratory study. Indian J Psychiatry 55(Suppl 3):S379–384

Hasani-Ranjbar S, Nayebi N, Larijani B et al (2009) A systematic review of the efficacy and safety of herbal medicines used in the treatment of obesity. World J Gastroenterol 15(25):3073–3085

Hemilä H, Chalker E (2013) Vitamin C for preventing and treating the common cold. Cochrane Database Syst Rev Jan 31;1:CD000980

Hershey AD, Powers SW, Vockell AL et al (2007) Coenzyme Q10 deficiency and response to supplementation in pediatric and adolescent migraine. Headache 47(1):73–80

Hiscock H, Scalzo K, Canterford L et al (2011) Sleep duration and body mass index in 0–7-year olds. Arch Dis Child 96(8):735

Ho M, Gow M, Halim J et al (2013) Effect of a prescriptive dietary intervention on psychological dimensions of eating behavior in obese adolescents. Int J Behav Nutr Phys Act 10(1):119

Hoelscher DM, Kirk S, Ritchie L, Academy Positions Committee (2013) Position of the Academy of Nutrition and Diabetics: interventions for the prevention and treatment of pediatric overweight and obesity. J Acad Nutr Diet 113(10):1375–1394

Holloway EA, West RJ (2007) Integrated breathing and relaxation training (the Papworth method) for adults with asthma in primary care: a randomised controlled trial. Thorax 62(12):1039–1042

Holroyd KA, Nash JM, Pingel JD et al (1991) A comparison of pharmacological (amitriptyline HCL) and nonpharmacological (cognitive-behavioral) therapies for chronic tension headaches. J Consult Clin Psychol 59(3):387–393

Houssen ME, Ragab A, Mesbah A et al (2010) Natural anti-inflammatory products and leukotriene inhibitors as complementary therapy for bronchial asthma. Clin Biochem 43(10–11):887–890

Hurt EA, Arnold LE, Lofthouse N (2011) Dietary and nutritional treatments for attention-deficit/ hyperactivity disorder: current research support and recommendations for practitioners. Curr Psychiatry Rep 13(5):323–332

ISH—International Headache Society, Headache Classification Subcommittee (2004) The international classification of headache disorders: 2nd edition. Cephalalgia 24(Suppl 1):9–160. (www .ihs-classification.org 10 Dec 2013)

Jaber R (2002) Respiratory and allergic diseases: from upper respiratory tract infections to asthma. Prim Care 29(2):231–261

Jensen ME, Gibson PG, Collins CE et al (2013) Diet-induced weight loss in obese children with asthma: a randomized controlled trial. Clin Exp Allergy 43(7):775–784

John PJ, Sharma N, Sharma CM et al (2007) Effectiveness of yoga therapy in the treatment of migraine without aura: a randomized controlled trial. Headache 47(5):654–661

Karlson G, Bennicke P (2013) Acupuncture in asthmatic children: a prospective, randomized, controlled clinical trial of efficacy. Altern Ther Health Med 19(4):13–19

Katz M, Levine AA, Kol-Degani H et al (2010) A compound herbal preparation (CHP) in the treatment of children with ADHD: a randomized controlled trial. J Atten Disord 14(3):281–291

Käufeler R, Polasek W, Brattström A et al (2006) Efficacy and safety of butterbur herbal extract Ze 339 in seasonal allergic rhinitis: postmarketing surveillance study. Adv Ther 23(2):373–384

Keen D, Hadijikoumi I (2011) ADHD in children and adolescents. Clin Evid (Online) 2011:pii: 0312

Kemper KJ (2002) The holistic pediatrician, 2nd edn. 1996 Harper Collins, New York. (Harper-Quill, 2002)

Khanam AA, Sachdeva U, Guleria R et al (1996) Study of pulmonary and autonomic functions of asthma patients after yoga training. Indian J Physiol Pharmacol 40(4):318–324

Kim S, Arora M, Fernandez C et al (2013) Lead, mercury, and cadmium exposure and attention deficit hyperactivity disorder in children. Environ Res 126:105–110

Konstantaki E, Priftis KN, Antonogeorgos G et al (2013) The association of sedentary lifestyle with childhood asthma. The role of nurse as educator. Allergol Immunopathol (Madr) pii: S0301–0546(13)00199–7

Krisanaprakornkit T, Ngamjarus C, Witoonchart C et al (2010) Meditation therapies for attention-deficit/hyperactivity disorder (ADHD). Cochrane Database Syst Rev Jun 16;(6):CD006507

Krouse JH, Krouse HJ (1999) Patient use of traditional and complementary therapies in treating rhinosinusitis before consulting an otolaryngologist. Laryngoscope 109(8):1223–1227

Kumari H, Pushpan R, Nishteswar K (2013) Medohara and Lekhaniya dravyas (anti-obesity and hypolipidemic drugs) in Ayurvedic classics: A critical review. Ayu 34(1):11–16

Ladomenou F, Kafatos A, Tselentis Y et al (2010) Predisposing factors for acute otitis media in infancy. J Infect 61(1):49

Lasisi AO (2009) The role of retinol in the etiology and outcome of suppurative otitis media. Eur Arch Otorhinolaryngol 266(5):647–652

Lee MS, Choi TY, Kim JI et al (2011) Acupuncture for treating attention deficit hyperactivity disorder: a systematic review and meta-analysis. Chin J Integr Med 17(4):257–260

Legarda SB, McMahon D, Othmer S et al (2011) Clinical neurofeedback: case studies, proposed mechanism, and implications for pediatric neurology practice. J Child Neurol 26(8):1045–1051

Lenon GB, Li CG, Da Costa C et al (2012) Lack of efficacy of a herbal preparation (RCM-102) for seasonal allergic rhinitis: a double blind, randomised, placebo-controlled trial. Asia Pac Allergy 2(3):187–194

Levi JR, Brody RM, McKee-Cole K et al (2013) Complementary and alternative medicine for pediatric otitis media. Int J Pediatr Otorhinolaryngol 77(6):926–931

Lewis DW, Yonker M, Winner P et al (2005) The treatment of pediatric migraine. Pediatr Ann 34:448–460

Li S, Yu B, Zhou D et al (2011) Acupuncture for attention deficit hyperactivity disorder (ADHD) in children and adolescents. Cochrane Database Syst Rev Apr 13;(4):CD007839

Lieberthal AS, Carroll AE, Chonmaitree T et al (2013) The diagnosis and management of acute otitis media. Pediatrics 131(3):e964–999

Linday LA (2010) Cod liver oil, young children, and upper respiratory tract infections. J Am Coll Nutr 29(6):559–562

Linday LA, Dolitsky JN, Shindledecker RD et al (2002) Lemon-flavored cod liver oil and a multivitamin-mineral supplement for the secondary prevention of otitis media in young children: pilot research. Ann Otol Rhinol Laryngol 111(7 Pt 1):642–652

Linday LA, Shindledecker RD, Dolitsky JN et al (2008) Plasma 25-hydroxyvitamin D levels in young children undergoing placement of tympanostomy tubes. Ann Otol Rhinol Laryngol 117(10):740–744

Linde K, Allais G, Brinkhaus B et al (2009) Acupuncture for migraine prophylaxis. Cochrane Database Syst Rev. Jan 21;(1):CD001218

Loder E, Burch R, Rizzoli P (2012) The 2012 AHS/AAN guidelines for prevention of episodic migraine: a summary and comparison with other recent clinical practice guidelines. Headache 52:930–945

Long KA, Ewing LJ, Cohen S et al (2011) Preliminary evidence for the feasibility of a stress management intervention for 7- to 12-year-olds with asthma. J Asthma 48(2):162–170

Loo EX, Llanora GV, Lu Q et al (2013) Supplementation with probiotics in the first 6 months of life did not protect against eczema and allergy in at-risk Asian infants: a 5-year follow-up. Int Arch Allergy Immunol 163(1):25–28

Madrid A, Rostel G, Pennington D et al (1995) Subjective assessment of allergy relief following group hypnosis and self-hypnosis: a preliminary study. Am J Clin Hypn 38(2):80–86

Maki KC, Davidson MH, Tsushima R et al (2002) Consumption of diacylglycerol oil as part of a reduced-energy diet enhances loss of body weight and fat in comparison with consumption of a triacylglycerol control oil. Am J Clin Nutr 76(6):1230–1236

Malik VS, Pan A, Willett WC et al (2013) Sugar-sweetened beverages and weight gain in children and adults: a systematic review and meta-analysis. Am J Clin Nutr 98(4):1084–1102

Manz F, Wentz A (2005) The importance of good hydration for the prevention of chronic diseases. Nutr Rev 63(6 Pt 2):S2–5

Marchisio P, Bianchini S, Galeone C et al (2011) Use of complementary and alternative medicine in children with recurrent acute otitis media in Italy. Int J Immunopathol Pharmacol 24(2):441–449

Mathie RT, Frye J, Fisher P (2012) Homeopathic Oscillococcinum(®) for preventing and treating influenza and influenza-like illness. Cochrane Database Syst Rev Dec 12;12:CD001957

Matkovic Z, Zivkovic V, Korica M et al (2010) Efficacy and safety of *Astragalus membranaceus* in the treatment of patients with seasonal allergic rhinitis. Phytother Res 24(2):175–181

McCrory DC, Williams JW, Dolor RJ et al (2003) Management of allergic rhinitis in the working-age population. Evid Rep Technol Assess (Summ) 67:1–4

Mehdi M, Farhad G, Alireza ME et al (2013) Comparison between the efficacy of ginger and sumatriptan in the ablative treatment of the common migraine. Phytother Res 28:412–415 doi:10.1002/ptr.4996. (Epub ahead of print)

Mehta S, Mehta V, Mehta S et al (2011) Multimodal behavior program for ADHD incorporating yoga and implemented by high school volunteers: a pilot study. ISRN Pediatr 2011:780745

Mehta S, Shah D, Shah K et al (2012) Peer-mediated multimodal intervention program for the treatment of children with ADHD in India: one-year followup. ISRN Pediatr 2012:419168

Meucci M, Cook C, Curry CD et al (2013) Effects of supervised exercise program on metabolic function in overweight adolescents. World J Pediatr 9(4):307–311

Migdow J (2013) Allergy antidote. http://www.yogajournal.com/health/885. Accessed 26 Dec 2013

Milan SJ, Hart A, Wilkinson M (2013) Vitamin C for asthma and exercise-induced bronchoconstriction. Cochrane Database Syst Rev Oct 23;10:CD010391

Miles EA, Calder PC (2014) Omega-6 and omega-3 polyunsaturated fatty acids and allergic diseases in infancy and childhood. Curr Pharm Des 20:946–953.

Millichap JG, Yee MM (2003) The diet factor in pediatric and adolescent migraine. Pediatr Neurol 28(1):9–15

Mims JW, Biddy AC (2013) Efficacy of environmental controls for inhalant allergies. Curr Opin Otolaryngol Head Neck Surg 21(3):241–247

Mitchell EA, Stewart AW, Clayton T et al (2009) Cross-sectional survey of risk factors for asthma in 6–7-year-old children in New Zealand: international study of asthma and allergy in childhood phase three. J Paediatr Child Health 45(6):375–383

Mitchell EA, Beasley R, Björkstén B, ISAAC phase three study group et al (2013) The association between BMI, vigorous physical activity and television viewing and the risk of symptoms of asthma, rhinoconjunctivitis and eczema in children and adolescents: ISAAC phase three. Clin Exp Allergy 43(1):73–84

Muir JM (2012) Chiropractic management of a patient with symptoms of attention-deficit/hyperactivity disorder. J Chiropr Med 11(3):221–224

Nestoriuc Y, Martin A (2007) Efficacy of biofeedback for migraine: a meta-analysis. Pain 128(1–2):111–127

NHBLI—National Heart, Blood, and Lung Institute (2007) Expert Panel Report 3 (EPR 3): guidelines for the diagnosis and management of asthma. NIH Publication no. 08–4051

Nicklas TA, O'Neil CE, Kleinman R (2008) Association between 100 % juice consumption and nutrient intake and weight in children aged 2–11 years. Arch Ped Adolesc Med 162:557–565

Nystad W, Håberg SE, London SJ et al (2008) Baby swimming and respiratory health. Acta Paediatr 97(5):657–662

O'Neil CE, Nicklas TA, Kleinman R (2010) Relationship between 100 % juice consumption and nutrient intake and weight of adolescents. Am J Health Promot 24:231–237

O'Neil CE, Nicklas TA, Rampersaud GC et al (2012) 100 % orange juice consumption is associated with better diet quality, improved nutrient adequacy, decreased risk for obesity, and improved biomarkers of health in adults: National Health and Nutrition Examination Survey, 2003–2006. Nutr J 11:107

Oelkers-Ax R, Leins A, Parzer P et al (2008) Butterbur root extract and music therapy in the prevention of childhood migraine: an explorative study. Eur J Pain 12(3):301–313

Ogden CL, Carroll MD, Kit BK, et al (2012) Prevalence of obesity in the United States, 2009–2010. NCHS data brief, no 82. Hyattsville, MD: National Center for Healt Statistics

Opat AJ, Cohen MM, Bailey MJ et al (2000) A clinical trial of the Buteyko breathing technique in asthma as taught by a video. J Asthma 37(7):557–564

Ozdemir O (2010) Any benefits of probiotics in allergic disorders? Allergy Asthma Proc 31(2):103–111

Patel SS, Beer S, Kearney DL et al (2013) Green tea extract: a potential cause of acute liver failure. World J Gastroenterol 19(31):5174–5177

Pattonder RK, Chandola HM, Vyas SN (2011) Clinical efficacy of Shilajatu (Asphaltum) processed with Agnimantha (Clerodendrum phlomidis Linn.) in Sthaulya (obesity). Ayu 32(4):526–531

Pellow J, Solomon EM, Barnard CN (2011) Complementary and alternative medical therapies for children with attention-deficit/hyperactivity disorder (ADHD). Altern Med Rev 16(4):323–337

Pelsser LM, Frankena K, Toorman J et al (2011) Effects of a restricted elimination diet on the behaviour of children with attention-deficit hyperactivity disorder (INCA study): a randomised controlled trial. Lancet 377(9764):494–503

Pendleton M, Brown S, Thomas C et al (2012) Potential toxicity of caffeine when used as a dietary supplement for weight loss. J Diet Suppl 9(4):293–298

Pepino VC, Ribeiro JD, Ribeiro MA et al (2013) Manual therapy for childhood respiratory disease: a systematic review. J Manipulative Physiol Ther 36(1):57–65

Pittler MH, Ernst E (2005) Complementary therapies for reducing body weight: a systematic review. Int J Obes (Lond) 29(9):1030–1038

Pohlman KA, Holton-Brown MS (2012) Otitis media and spinal manipulative therapy: a literature review. J Chiropr Med 11(3):160–169

Posadzki P, Lee MS, Ernst E (2013) Osteopathic manipulative treatment for pediatric conditions: a systematic review. Pediatrics 132(1):140–152

Pothmann R, Danesch U (2005) Migraine prevention in children and adolescents: results of an open study with a special butterbur root extract. Headache 45(3):196–203

Prescott SL, Tang ML (2005) The Australasian Society of Clinical Immunology and allergy position statement: summary of allergy prevention in children. Med J Aust 182(9):464–467

Rajan TV, Tennen H, Lindquist RL et al (2002) Effect of ingestion of honey on symptoms of rhinoconjunctivitis. Ann Allergy Asthma Immunol 88(2):198–203

Ramchandani NM (2010) Homeopathic treatment of upper respiratory tract infections in children: evaluation of thirty case series. Complement Ther Clin Pract 16(2):101–108

Reinhold T, Roll S, Willich SN et al (2013) Cost-effectiveness for acupuncture in seasonal allergic rhinitis: economic results of the ACUSAR trial. Ann Allergy Asthma Immunol 111(1):56–63

Rommel AS, Halperin JM, Mill J et al (2013) Protection from genetic diathesis in attention-deficit/hyperactivity disorder: possible complementary roles of exercise. J Am Acad Child Adolesc Psychiatry 52(9):900–910

Rommelse N, Buitelaar J (2013) Is there a future for restricted elimination diets in ADHD clinical practice? Eur Child Adolesc Psychiatry 22(4):199–202

Rosenkranz RR, Rosenkranz SK, Neessen KJ (2012) Dietary factors associated with lifetime asthma or hayfever diagnosis in Australian middle-aged and older adults: a cross-sectional study. Nutr J 11:84

Rosenlund H, Magnusson J, Kull I et al (2012) Antioxidant intake and allergic disease in children. Clin Exp Allergy 42(10):1491–1500

Russell H (2013) Allergy antidote. http://www.yogajournal.com/health/885. Accessed 26 Dec 2013

Saadeh D, Salameh P, Baldi I et al (2013) Diet and allergic diseases among population aged 0–18 years: myth or reality? Nutrients 5(9):3399–3423

Saarinen K, Jantunen J, Haahtela T (2011) Birch pollen honey for birch pollen allergy–a randomized controlled pilot study. Int Arch Allergy Immunol 155(2):160–166

Sarrell EM, Cohen HA, Kahan E (2003) Naturopathic treatment for ear pain in children. Pediatrics 111:E574–E579

Sarrell EM, Mandelberg A, Cohen HA (2001) Efficacy of naturopathic extracts in the management of ear pain associated with acute otitis media. Arch Pediatr Adolesc Med 155:796–799

Sarris J, Kean J, Schweitzer I et al (2011) Complementary medicines (herbal and nutritional products) in the treatment of attention deficit hyperactivity disorder (ADHD): a systematic review of the evidence. Complement Ther Med 19(4):216–227

Saxena VS, Venkateshwarlu K, Nadig P et al (2004) Multicenter clinical trials on a novel polyherbal formulation in allergic rhinitis. Int J Clin Pharmacol Res 24(2–3):79–94

Schiapparelli P, Allais G, Castagnoli Gabellari I et al (2010) Non-pharmacological approach to migraine prophylaxis: part II. Neurol Sci 31(Suppl 1):S137–139

Schlotz W, Jones A, Phillips DI et al (2010) Lower maternal folate status in early pregnancy is associated with childhood hyperactivity and peer problems in offspring. J Child Psychol Psychiatry 51(5):594–602

Science M, Maguire JL, Russell ML et al (2013) Low serum 25-hydroxyvitamin D level and risk of upper respiratory tract infection in children and adolescents. Clin Infect Dis 57(3):392–397

Seida JK, Durec T, Kuhle S (2011) North American (Panax quinquefolius) and Asian Ginseng (Panax ginseng) preparations for prevention of the common cold in healthy adults: a systematic review. Evid Based Complement Alternat Med 2011:282151

Seo JH, Kwon SO, Lee SY et al (2013) Association of antioxidants with allergic rhinitis in children from seoul. Allergy Asthma Immunol Res 5(2):81–87

Shah UH, Kalra V (2009) Pediatric migraine. Int J Pediatr 2009:424192

Singhal HK, Neetu, Kumar A et al (2010) Ayurvedic approach for improving reaction time of attention deficit hyperactivity disorder affected children. Ayu 31(3):338–342

Sioen I, Den Hond E, Nelen V et al (2013) Prenatal exposure to environmental contaminants and behavioural problems at age 7–8 years. Environ Int 59:225–231

Skoner DP (2001) Allergic rhinitis: definition, epidemiology, pathophysiology, detection, and diagnosis. J Allergy Clin Immunol 108(suppl 1):S2–S8

Slater SK, Nelson TD, Kabbouche MA et al (2011) A randomized, double-blinded, placebo-controlled, crossover, add-on study of CoEnzyme Q10 in the prevention of pediatric and adolescent migraine. Cephalalgia 31(8):897–905

Sonuga-Barke EJ, Brandeis D, Cortese S et al (2013) European ADHD guidelines group. Non-pharmacological interventions for ADHD: systematic review and meta-analyses of randomized controlled trials of dietary and psychological treatments. Am J Psychiatry 170(3):275–289

Stevens LJ, Kuczek T, Burgess JR et al (2011) Dietary sensitivities and ADHD symptoms: thirty-five years of research. Clin Pediatr (Phila) 50(4):279–293

Steyer TE, Ables A (2009) Complementary and alternative therapies for weight loss. Prim Care 36(2):395–406

Stoelzel K, Bothe G, Chong PW et al (2013) Safety and efficacy of Nasya/Prevalin in reducing symptoms of allergic rhinitis. Clin Respir J. 2013 Nov 27. doi: 10.1111/crj.12080. (Epub ahead of print)

Strachan DP, Cook DG (1998) Health effects of passive smoking.4. Parental smoking, middle ear disease and adenotonsillectomy in children. Thorax 53(1):50–56

Torres-Llenza V, Bhogal S, Davis M, Ducharme F (2010) Use of complementary and alternative medicine in children with asthma. Can Respir J 17(4):183–187

TPS—Texas Pediatrics Society (2013) Texas Pediatrics Society. http://txpeds.org/obesity-toolkit-resources. Accessed 1 Jan 2014

Trasande L, Attina TM, Blustein J (2012) Association between urinary bisphenol A concentration and obesity prevalence in children and adolescents. JAMA 308(11):1113

Uhari M, Mäntysaari K, Niemelä M (1996) A meta-analytic review of the risk factors for acute otitis media. Clin Infect Dis 22(6):1079–1083

Vlachojannis JE, Cameron M, Chrubasik S (2010) A systematic review on the sambuci fructus effect and efficacy profiles. Phytother Res 24(1):1–8

Vohra S, Johnston BC, Laycock KL et al (2008) Safety and tolerability of North American ginseng extract in the treatment of pediatric upper respiratory tract infection: a phase II randomized, controlled trial of 2 dosing schedules. Pediatrics 122(2):e402–410

Wahl RA, Aldous MB, Worden KA (2008) Echinacea purpurea and osteopathic manipulative treatment in children with recurrent otitis media: a randomized controlled trial. BMC Complement Altern Med 8:56

Wald ER (2005) To treat or not to treat. Pediatrics 115(4):1087

Wang F, Van Den Eeden SK, Ackerson LM et al (2003) Oral magnesium oxide prophylaxis of frequent migrainous headache in children: a randomized, double-blind, placebo-controlled trial. Headache 43(6):601–610

Wang MC, Liu CY, Shiao AS et al (2005) Ear problems in swimmers. J Chin Med Assoc 68(8):347–352

Wang B, Lei F, Cheng G (2007) Acupuncture treatment of obesity with magnetic needles–a report of 100 cases. J Tradit Chin Med 27(1):26–27

Wang H, Li W, Ju XF et al (2013) Effect of penetrating needling at head acupoints on perennial allergic rhinitis. Zhongguo Zhen Jiu 33(9):789–792. (Article in Chinese)

Weber W, Taylor JA, Stoep AV et al (2005) Echinacea purpurea for prevention of upper respiratory tract infections in children. J Altern Complement Med 11(6):1021–1026

WebMD (2013) Natural allergy relief. http://www.webmd.com/allergies/features/natural-allergy-relief. Accessed 27 Dec 2013

Yang YQ, Chen HP, Wang Y et al (2013) Considerations for use of acupuncture as supplemental therapy for patients with allergic asthma. Clin Rev Allergy Immunol 44(3):254–261

Yao TC, Chang CJ, Hsu YH et al (2010) Probiotics for allergic diseases: realities and myths. Pediatr Allergy Immunol 21(6):900–919

Yu C, Zhao S, Zhao X (1998) Treatment of simple obesity in children with photo-acupuncture. Zhongguo Zhong Xi Yi Jie He Za Zhi 18(6):348–50. (Article in Chinese)

Zhang H, Peng Y, Liu Z et al (2011) Effects of acupuncture therapy on abdominal fat and hepatic fat content in obese children: a magnetic resonance imaging and proton magnetic resonance spectroscopy study. J Altern Complement Med 17(5):413–420

Zhu S, Wang N, Wang D et al (1998) A clinical investigation on massage for prevention and treatment of recurrent respiratory tract infection in children. J Tradit Chin Med 18(4):285–291

Zutavern A, Brockow I, Schaaf B et al (2008) LISA Study Group. Timing of solid food introduction in relation to eczema, asthma, allergic rhinitis, and food and inhalant sensitization at the age of 6 years: results from the prospective birth cohort study LISA. Pediatrics 121(1):e44–52

Chapter 5
The Future of Integrative Pediatrics

Sanghamitra M. Misra

Integrative pediatrics is a quickly developing field due to demand from the patient population. As CAM modalities become increasingly popular, general pediatric practitioners bear the burden of becoming knowledgeable about CAM medicines and therapies. Although the vast majority of pediatric providers will not specialize in integrative pediatrics, all pediatric providers need a basic understanding of the various types of medicine and therapies available to their patients. This knowledge is vital to protecting and guiding pediatric patients and their families. As the body of literature grows, effective therapies will be utilized more frequently and less effective therapies will be utilized less frequently. With time, it is possible that all of pediatrics will be considered integrative pediatrics with a focus on mind, body, and spirit and with a concept of utilizing all effective therapies, allopathic and non-allopathic, for the good of the patient.

S. M. Misra (✉)
Academic General Pediatrics, Baylor College of Medicine, Houston, TX, USA
email: smisra@bcm.edu

S. M. Misra, A. Maria Verissimo, *A Guide to Integrative Pediatrics for the Healthcare Professional,* SpringerBriefs in Public Health, DOI 10.1007/978-3-319-06835-0_5,   95
© Springer International Publishing Switzerland 2014

Index

Printed in the United States
By Bookmasters